RASĀYANA

GEETA VARA

RASĀYANA

FEEL YOUNG *in* MIND AND BODY *with* *the* WISDOM *of* ĀYURVEDA

GREEN TREE
LONDON • OXFORD • NEW YORK • NEW DELHI • SYDNEY

GREEN TREE
Bloomsbury Publishing Plc
50 Bedford Square, London, WC1B 3DP, UK
Bloomsbury Publishing Ireland Limited,
29 Earlsfort Terrace, Dublin 2, D02 AY28, Ireland

BLOOMSBURY, GREEN TREE and the Green Tree logo are trademarks of Bloomsbury Publishing Plc

First published in Great Britain 2026

A catalogue record for this book is available from the British Library.

Library of Congress Cataloguing-in-Publication data has been applied for.

ISBN: PB: 978-1-3994-2980-1; eBook: 978-1-3994-2981-8; ePDF: 978-1-3994-2979-5

2 4 6 8 10 9 7 5 3 1

Illustrations on pp. 46, 68, 97, 166–71 and 178 by Barking Dog Art
Typeset in Avenir Next by Lumina Datamatics Ltd

Printed and bound in Great Britain by Clays Ltd, Elcograf S.p.A

FSC www.fsc.org
MIX
Paper | Supporting responsible forestry
FSC® C018072

To find out more about our authors and books visit www.bloomsbury.com and sign up for our newsletters.

For product safety related questions contact productsafety@bloomsbury.com

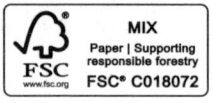

लोकाः समस्ताः सुखिनो भवन्तु

Lokāḥ Samastāḥ Sukhino Bhavantu

May all beings everywhere be happy and free

Contents

How to use this book

This book unfolds in two parts, designed to gently guide your journey of pro-ageing through the wisdom of *rasāyana*, *Āyurveda* and the wider Vedic traditions.

- **Part 1** lays the foundations – the philosophy, principles and inner workings of *Āyurveda* and *rasāyana*. We explore how the body ages and how the soul grows, along with essential cleansing preparations and why they matter for ageing well.
- **Part 2** explores the **seven pillars of pro-ageing** and offers practical, everyday ways to nourish body, mind and spirit.

It's always most enriching when you read a book from start to finish, but you can also dip into any section that calls to you and come back to it at any time as a source of reference.

A note on terminology

Rasāyana can mean many things at once. In this book, when we use the term '*rasāyana*' it may refer to a medicine made of rejuvenating herbs; a therapy that restores vitality; a lifestyle that supports balance; a philosophy of adding life to years; and a spiritual path that nourishes the soul. It can be a technique, such as living with truth, compassion and calm; a tool to preserve ***ojas*** (our subtle vitality); or a way of restoring inner balance and strength. For me, it's the original pro-ageing system, one that promotes longevity and vitality in every sense. In essence, *rasāyana* is anything that helps you feel renewed in mind, body and mood – whether it's a herb, a thought, a ritual or a way of being.

In this book, I use the term ***Āyurveda*** to refer to the wider science of life beyond the specific branch of *rasāyana*.

Pro-ageing is the art of growing older with grace – not fighting time but flowing with it. It's about nourishing the mind and body, honouring change and allowing wisdom to gently navigate growth. Pro-ageing means ageing consciously reflected through our daily choices, welcoming time as a teacher and living deeply.

Pro-ageing embraces ageing as a positive process. It is a mindset of joyful acceptance and a philosophy to live by, growing with wisdom. *Rasāyana* is the original pro-ageing system – designed to keep our essence (***rasa***) flowing strongly through every season of life.

Vitality, in simple terms, is vibrant health – the energy, awareness and joy that make us feel fully alive. In *Āyurveda*, this vitality is sustained by optimising *ojas* (resilience), ***tejas*** (radiance) and ***prāṇa*** (life force). It's the steady glow that comes from inner balance and deep nourishment. Vitality is what expands our healthspan – the years we live with strength, clarity and purpose.

The **'vitality gap'** refers in this book to the difference between how long we live and how well we live – when lifespan outlasts healthspan. Closing this gap is at the heart of *rasāyana* and pro-ageing: a quest to sustain vitality throughout life's changing seasons.

A note on Sanskrit and pronunciation

Throughout this book, you'll find **Sanskrit** words written in italics using diacritic marks (IAST) to preserve accuracy in pronunciation and to honour their original form. This approach helps preserve the integrity of key *Āyurvedic* and **Vedic** terms such as *rasāyana*, *prāṇa* and ***doṣas***.

A small line above a vowel (ā, ī, ū) means you hold the sound a little longer – *rasāyana becomes rasaa-yana, pronounced* Rah-SAA-Yah-Nuh*;* *prāṇa* becomes 'praa-nuh', the breath that sustains life. A tiny dot beneath certain letters (ṣ, ṭ, ḍ, ṇ) means you pronounce them with the tongue curled slightly back, giving *doṣa* its soft 'shh' sound, pronounced as 'doh-sha'.

A glossary of key words is provided at the end of the book to help you understand the literal translation more easily. Words included in the glossary are highlighted in bold when first introduced in the text.

Introduction

For as long as we've walked this earth, humans have chased the idea of staying young. We're constantly seeking that elusive formula for vitality, yet many of us live in ways that inadvertently drain our energy and accelerate ageing.

We are all a little bit (or maybe a lot) burnt out from the multiple demands of modern life, particularly in the urban jungles. Somehow, we have become accustomed to this, and even idolise the work hard, play hard model of living. Push harder, run faster, do more, achieve more, simultaneously facing social, financial, work and relationship pressures. This is having a detrimental effect on our well-being and how we age.

Interestingly, the World Health Organization (WHO) says we are now living longer than ever. By 2020, the number of people aged 60 years and older outnumbered children younger than five years. With this increase in lifespan has come a rise in age-related conditions – many of which were less common in earlier eras. In effect, we're living longer than ever, but not necessarily better.

So far, we've become skilled at prolonging life, but not at extending the years that feel vibrant and clear. This has created what I call a 'vitality gap', the space between the length of our lives and the quality of those extra years. Too often that 'gap' is spent in decline, managing chronic illness or frailty.

We may feel invincible in our 20s and 30s, with bags of energy, rarely stopping (or wanting) to think about the deeper process of ageing until it catches up with us later on. But instead of waiting for old age to bring its challenges, what if we chose to invest in our health like a pension scheme, paid into day by day?

It's time to shift our focus towards truly future-proofing ourselves and invest in the habits and practices that will help us live those added years with vitality. This is the key focus of this book: 'pro-ageing' – not resisting ageing, but sustaining quality of life as we mature, through the timeless wisdom of *rasāyana*, the science of rejuvenation.

Rooted in *Āyurveda*, *rasāyana* offers a path to nurture vitality, extend healthspan and age with grace in body and mind. True pro-ageing isn't about chasing metrics or extending time at any cost – it's about delaying and preventing age-related decline through the daily choices we make in diet, lifestyle and environment. Our real work is to reduce the years lived in poor health, and enjoy more years in vibrancy, clarity and joy. The true measure of our health isn't just how long we live, but how fully and freely we can live every day.

Challenging accepted norms

We have been conditioned to equate ageing with decline, laced with disease, frailty, pain, loss of energy, diminished mental sharpness and waning enthusiasm. Yet, around the world, we see communities, from Okinawa to Sardinia, flourishing well into their 90s and beyond, proving that decline is not the only story of ageing.

So, should we simply accept our bleak outlook as inevitable? This collective mindset needs to be challenged and redirected. Our beliefs, thoughts and actions deeply influence the trajectory of our ageing process. What if I said ageing didn't have to follow this downward spiral? What if we learned *how* to live? I mean to truly live, not merely exist, giving us the possibility of reaching 100, disease-free, with full mental acuity and physical vitality? Avoiding disease is not the goal, it's the side effect of living in a state of optimal well-being for our health today *and* for our future self.

Despite our rapid technological advancements, human biology hasn't evolved at the same pace. We have drifted from the way nature intended us to live, eating fast food instead of from the earth, sitting instead of squatting to poop and scrolling instead of sleeping. This growing disparity between how we live and how we're designed to thrive lies at the heart of our modern health crisis. Recognising this, many are turning to ancestral healing and ancient wisdom not from nostalgia, but to reclaim our original blueprint of vitality.

The modern wellness culture has become reliant on shortcuts. Chasing health trends and hacks, from extreme workouts to high-tech skin treatments promising youthful looks and instant results. But the unsexy truth is that these trends often yield only short-term results, rarely creating lasting well-being because they treat symptoms, not the whole human system.

What's more, we have been conditioned to believe that good health must be costly. But in reality, it begins with awareness and alignment, not products or pills. Can we *afford* to continue this trajectory? It's time to tune out from the noise and tune into the 'self'. It's time to get educated, aligned and aware, not 'influenced'. And this is where *rasāyana* enters the arena with a timeless path that transforms ageing into the art of renewal.

A short overview of *Āyurveda*

Āyurveda is not a passing wellness trend: it is, in many ways, the original longevity science, profoundly adaptable yet rooted in timeless traditions. It is the oldest known system of health and healing emerging from the Indian subcontinent, a living tradition that continues to guide us today. Rather than dividing the body into systems as modern medicine often does, *Āyurveda* views health as one interconnected whole – body, mind, spirit and environment.

At its heart, *Āyurveda* isn't about rigid rules or metrics but about living in tune with nature, through relationship, ritual and respect. It doesn't ask us to just 'follow a diet' or 'take a pill': it invites us to remember who we are – and teaches us how to align to that rhythm. It is both a deeply personalised system of medicine and philosophical guide to life. Its approach is both preventive and restorative, treating the root causes of imbalance while strengthening resilience. In a world of constant change, getting the basics right – food, breath, rest, connection – matters more today than ever.

The literal translation of *Āyurveda* is 'knowledge of life' (*āyu* = life, *veda* = knowledge). Born from *Āyurveda*'s body of timeless wisdom is *rasāyana, the* branch dedicated to rejuvenation supporting longevity, vitality and youthfulness.

प्रयोजनं चास्य स्वस्थस्य स्वास्थ्यरक्षणमातुरस्य ।
विकारप्रशमनं च ॥

prayojanaṃ cāsya svasthasya syāsthya rakṣaṇam, |
āturasya vikāra praśamanam ca ||

'The purpose of *Āyurveda* is to preserve the health of the healthy and to alleviate disease in the sick.'

Caraka Saṃhitā, Sūtrasthāna. 30.26

Āyurveda guides us to live in harmony with nature, to adapt to seasonal changes and to align with the cycles of the sun and moon, always respecting our unique mind–body constitutions (***prakṛti***).

Over my 20+ years of practice, I've seen more and more people grow frustrated with conventional 'medical fixes', sensing their health challenges stem from much deeper roots. Despite being 5000 years old, *Āyurveda* still holds the power to reshape our reality of ageing, disease and what it means to live well.

According to *Āyurveda*, our well-being is shaped not only by our genetics but also by our choices, histories (as far back as our mother's pregnancy) and even the mental–emotional patterns we inherit. True holistic healing is not disease-focused but always person-centred and multilayered in approach – through food, lifestyle, herbs, breath, meditation, movement, **mantras**, ***mudrās*** and a conscious relationship with our environment.

What the sages (known as ***Ṛṣi*** **(Rishi)** and ***Ācārya*** in Sanksrit) understood intuitively is being confirmed today through modern science, through fields such as quantum physics, neuroplasticity, nutrigenomics and functional medicine. We are learning that true health is dynamic, adaptable and deeply personal. *Āyurveda* stands strong as a living science: timeless and always relevant.

The history and journey of *Āyurveda*

This wisdom of *Āyurveda* is rooted in the **Vedas**, India's oldest body of knowledge (c. 1500–500 BCE), which explore ritual, philosophy and the nature of existence. Out of this tapestry, alongside sister sciences **yoga**, ***vastu*** (the Vedic science of dwelling and space) and ***jyotiṣa*** (astrology), *Āyurveda* emerged as a practical system for health and longevity. Some believe it was received by sages (*Ṛṣis*) through deep meditation and passed down orally; others resonate with the story of Lord Dhanvantari rising from the cosmic ocean with the nectar of immortality (*amṛta*) and the teachings of *Āyurveda*. Both routes show us that this knowledge has always been seen as sacred, linking human life with the rhythms of the cosmos.

Preserved for centuries in classical texts such as the *Caraka Saṃhitā, Suśruta Saṃhitā* and ***Aṣṭāṅga Hṛdaya***, *Āyurveda* nearly disappeared under the British colonisation of India, but survived through oral traditions, Sanskrit verses and lived practice. Today, it has found a renewed relevance, both as a system of medicine and a guide for prevention of disease, vitality and longevity.

Rasāyana – the science of rejuvenation

Rasāyana, one of *Āyurveda*'s eight branches, translates as 'the science of resilience, rejuvenation and longevity' or, as I like to call it, the Āyurvedic art of 'maturing with grace'. Biological ageing is inevitable, but through the wisdom of *rasāyana,* we can slow the ageing process and mitigate related health issues by addressing the root causes.

For me, spirituality and science are not separate but deeply intertwined – and *rasāyana* is the gateway between them. When we cultivate strength in the body and steadiness in the mind, we free up energy to live our purpose, expand in wisdom and grow spiritually. Health, then, is not the final goal: it is the foundation for a joyful, meaningful and fulfilling life.

Popular wellness trends often take a reductionist approach focusing on detoxification, clean eating, fasting and cleansing. We often hear

'I'm on a detox' or 'I'm on a diet,' which can be useful for recalibrating our short-term health but when it comes to longevity (lifespan) and vitality (healthspan), the real question is, how are you future-proofing your long-term health?

Āyurveda sees cleansing practices as essential but just a *part* of a larger framework of healing. Pro-ageing is not limited to cleansing, but about deep nourishment for the body, mind and spirit. This deep nourishment sits at the heart of *rasāyana*: strengthening the mind and body to build resilience and vitality – the essence of immunity as we understand it today. *Rasāyana* therapy enhances vital energy (*ojas*), strengthens immunity and aligns your life with your soul's truth. It blends rejuvenation and gentle detoxification through tailored nutrition, herbal tonics, movement, mindset and spiritual awareness to sustain long-term health.

In my first book, *Ayurveda: Ancient Wisdom for Modern Wellbeing*, I focused on a personalised approach to health based on *prakṛti* (our unique mind–body constitution) with a deep dive into gut health, balancing *doṣas* through rituals and routine. In this book, I draw from the same roots of *Āyurvedic* wisdom while taking the conversation in a new direction of slowing our biological ageing and preventing its associated conditions through ancient insights.

In the coming pages, I'll introduce you to the wisdom and principles of *Āyurveda* and *rasāyana* embedded in Vedic philosophy and what it means to embrace ageing. We dive deep into the practical and profound tools that can help you reclaim vitality and age with grace in our current climate through the seven pillars of pro-ageing in part 2.

Ageing is not a disease but the process of life itself. We can choose how we experience it: either as a slow decline or as an opportunity to cultivate vitality, wisdom and joy. Regardless of your age, your choices today and onwards will influence how you age, and I hope the writings of this book help keep your biological age younger than your chronological age.

A note on understanding Āyurveda

Āyurveda is not a one-size-fits-all framework, but a personalised and experiential system of healing. It's therefore helpful to move through this book with openness and curiosity for its nuanced approach to understanding the mind-body. When *Āyurveda's* lived practices observed over centuries are evaluated through the Western medical or experimental lens, it can feel like trying to fit a square peg into a round hole. It's promising that many *Āyurvedic* principles and practices have growing scientific support, but the value of its wisdom should not depend on that validation alone.

My personal journey

Since writing my first book on *Āyurveda*, *rasāyana* has become central to both my work and how I live, especially as I navigate my own health changes. By my late-30s, I began noticing subtle but unsettling shifts in my health. My energy wasn't the same. I was shedding more hair, finding more silver strands, and my skin had lost its glow. I was becoming forgetful, sleeping poorly and feeling dizzy for no clear reason. These weren't dramatic illnesses that I felt warranted a visit to the GP or needed medical tests, but they were signals from my body, hinting at deeper imbalances and, perhaps if I am honest, premature ageing. Conventional medicine didn't have much to offer for these 'in-between' spaces – where you're not sick, but you're far from thriving. *Āyurveda*, on the other hand, takes such early signs seriously, treating them as opportunities to restore balance before decline sets in. It became the turning point to deepen the practice of what I preach!

I was already living *Āyurveda*, so it wasn't about adding more to my to-do list. Instead, it was about going deeper, becoming more consistent, honouring the right changes for my mind-body type and even softening some of my ego-driven desires so I could prioritise differently. I began to bring *Āyurveda*'s rejuvenation branch, *rasāyana*, to the forefront. This included steady routines, seasonal alignment, *rasāyana* herbs and recipes, and deep rest, consciously weaving in practices that nourish both mind and body into my daily life.

Today, I am certainly feeling younger and more vibrant than my trips around the sun suggest and the tools I share in this book are the same ones I continue to live by and a reflection of how I work with my clients.

Growing up in the UK, I saw first-hand how migration reshaped my family's way of living. Like many Indian migrants, my parents had to adapt quickly, juggling the strains of survival, fitting in to a new culture and managing without familiar foods, essential comforts and community support. Despite holding onto cultural practices, over time and without realising, Western habits replaced Indian traditions – habits that felt modern but eroded health, especially with exposure to packaged and fast foods. Today, within the South Asian community abroad, I see the cost: lifestyle-related illnesses rising and long lists of daily prescriptions now accepted as 'normal'.

In the move across oceans for greener pastures, something precious slipped away: the way we ate, the way we lived, the way we understood health and family closeness. And now, I see that same erosion unfolding in my motherland, India. As an *Āyurvedic* practitioner, this both saddens and fuels me. I often think, *I want my cupboard to be filled with food, not pharma*.

As a first-generation British-born Indian, I grew up between two contrasting cultures which at the time felt like an impossible feat. *Āyurveda* was present every day in countless small ways within my family, but it wasn't until I formally studied it that I understood how profoundly this wisdom speaks to the challenges of modern life. My path to this work began with my own process of reconnecting with my heritage, and today I help others understand themselves through the lens of *Āyurveda*, offering personalised guidance that includes diet, lifestyle, herbal support, emotional balance and self-evolution. My work with *Āyurveda* is for Western seekers and the global community but also to help South Asians – at home and abroad – reconnect with the richness of what we've been fortunate to inherit.

All of my grandparents have now left this earth. My Nani lived to 93, but her final years were shadowed by dementia – a painful reminder of why this work matters to me so deeply, and why, when it comes to preserving health, if we wait, it's already too late.

After writing my first book, I realised how deeply conditioned we are to the 'disease-focused' and 'fix-it' mindset, even within natural and Eastern healing systems, because we want to *see* and *feel* results now. And for most of us, if we are honest, we wait until something goes wrong before we pay attention. We need a paradigm shift from 'fix what's broken' to 'holistic healing' – a process that often requires the conscious undoing, unravelling and unlearning of deeply embedded habits and patterns. Let's use this book to remind ourselves of what preventative and optimal health really means and that we can never regret investing in and protecting our future selves.

Time to trust again

The seed for this book was planted in early 2020, at the start of the pandemic, when my intuition told me this work was needed, but divine timing had its own plan for its fruition. Perhaps I needed to be closer to my half-centenarian stage of life, or the world wasn't ready yet.

As this book comes to life in 2026, it carries even deeper meaning. It reflects my personal growth and the universal truth that some seeds take time to germinate, and we must trust the process. Trust and surrender are a tender life lesson. So, I am thrilled this book is finally born to the world because *rasāyana* itself is about acceptance, growth and trust in nature's timing.

As you read this book, I don't ask you to trust in me, but to trust in yourself – your body, your intuition, your soul's guidance, time and the lessons from nature.

Is *rasāyana* for you?

Absolutely! *Rasāyana* is for everyone. Whether you're recovering from burnout, healing after illness, feeling the weight of stress or simply wanting to feel more vibrant and resilient, *rasāyana* offers a gentle, intelligent way to age.

In the classical *Āyurvedic* texts, *rasāyana* was recommended for:

- Those recovering from long-term stress or disease
- People moving through seasonal transitions or life stage shifts
- The elderly wanting to age gracefully
- Children needing nourishment for healthy growth
- Expectant mothers building strength and vitality
- And anyone who has completed a detox or ***pañcakarma*** and wants to rebuild.

In truth, everyone can benefit from integrating *rasāyana*. If you're juggling deadlines, parenting, running a business or navigating the pace of modern life, you're likely using energy faster than you replenish it. *Rasāyana* helps you refill your cup so you can expand your healthspan and lifespan.

It's never too late or too early to be in the driving seat of your well-being. The sooner we build awareness, the more powerfully we can influence our biological age. You've heard the saying: 'The best time to start was yesterday. The second-best time is today'. Whether you're 20 or 70, you can choose to strengthen your body, sharpen your mind and nourish your soul. This isn't about resisting ageing: it's about embracing it fully and consciously. This is pro-ageing!

Part 1

The ancient wisdom of ageing well

1

The challenges of ageing

'All the powers in the universe are already ours. It is we who have put our hands before our eyes and cry that it is dark.'

Swami Vivekānanda

Old age is not a distant destination. Ageing is a journey that begins the minute we are born and something that unfolds gradually in its own time, *through* us rather than happening *to* us. You'll come to see how ancient *Āyurvedic* wisdom is receiving confirmation by modern science on the same truths: vitality and longevity aren't simply an accident of genetics or luck, but the result of how we live, think and connect.

Let's open the conversation in this chapter by exploring:

- Our fears around ageing
- The findings of my personal research
- How ageing shows up in the body and mind
- What causes ageing to accelerate.

Redefining ageing: from anti-ageing to pro-ageing

Much of what we experience as 'ageing' is largely steered by culture, internal beliefs and expressed attitudes, so perhaps the essential shift we need to make is reevaluating how we *relate* to ageing itself.

What is the story of your life? Every life story is essentially shaped by the choices that we make; and our healthspan is determined by how we show up for ourselves.

Let's be clear on one thing: ageing is *not* a disease. It is a natural, inevitable part of being alive, yet our culture often teaches us to fear and fight it. We are constantly bombarded with the term 'anti-ageing', but what does that really mean? Is youthfulness about staying wrinkle-free? Clinging to the illusion of being 20 forever?

Anti-ageing literally means 'resisting getting older' – something we all know is not possible in reality. Conversely, pro-ageing is about living longer *and* better – not fighting time but flowing with it. We're talking about being the healthiest and happiest version of ourselves at each stage of life. The focus of *Rasāyana* is on enhancing vitality, clarity, resilience and closing the 'vitality gap' between how long we live and how well we live. Recognising that we have total agency to rewrite our life story no matter our starting point is the biggest flex in life, especially when we embrace ageing with sovereignty.

What we really think and feel about ageing

Āyurveda may give us guiding principles, but what about our lived experience? Before I began writing this book, I wanted to hear those personal voices too. I ran a small exploratory and independent survey of adults from my personal and professional community grouped by age (under-60s and over-60s). It wasn't a large-scale study (perhaps one day it will be) but it gave meaningful insights that I've woven into these pages.

Your life story so far is part of the wider picture of what it means to age with awareness. So, perhaps *you* might like to pause for 10–15 minutes and reflect on the questions below as a way of checking in with your health, habits and mindset as we embark on the path of pro-ageing.

If you are under 60:

- How do you feel about ageing? Does it stir any emotions, images or concerns, or perhaps it feels like a natural process to embrace?
- Are your health choices more about the present moment or do you also consider your future self?

- How much do natural remedies and preventative practices matter to you?
- When you think of ageing, do you see it as an opportunity for growth, or as a set of hurdles?
- How much weight do you give to genetics compared to the daily habits you practise now?
- What about the influence of culture, values or social messages – whose voices do you hear when you imagine your later years? Are there elders you admire who show you what ageing well can look like?
- Are there aspects of the ageing process that feel especially empowering, or limiting?

If you are over 60:

- What has your lived experience of ageing been so far?
- Have changes arrived gradually or more suddenly?
- Are there things you wish you had done differently, or practices you would have adopted earlier to support your health?
- If you're thriving, what has helped you most – lifestyle, natural remedies, preventative practices or a deep sense of purpose?
- How have culture, family or community shaped your journey?
- Do you find ageing has opened more space for wisdom and growth, or has it felt more like a physical and mental challenge?
- And if you could, what advice would you offer your younger self, or the next generation, about embracing this process with grace?

These reflections highlight a simple truth: ageing is not just about adding years to life, but about the quality of those years. This is where the distinction between lifespan and healthspan becomes vital – the 'vitality gap'! The natural phase of ageing as we get older is referred to as ***Jarāvasthā***.

Learning and reflection: what participants said

Among participants over 60, 94 per cent said they would offer advice to their younger selves. The strongest message? *Start caring for your health earlier* – for your body, mind and relationships. Many wished they had practised more self-compassion, less perfectionism and better health education over career or material success.

But ageing also brought gifts. It was often described as a time of softening, moving with more acceptance of physical limitations, letting go of comparison and finding peace in who they are. Several found new strength in practices like *Āyurveda*, where rhythm, simple food habits, more rest, gentle movement and nature restored balance.

In my research, several women over 60 described feeling invisible as they age, due to ageism and appearance-based pressure. Menopause, body changes and shifting social values marginalise older women. And yet, these same women also spoke of discovering freedom, self-assurance and joy, proving that a new story is possible.

Most survey respondents believed lifestyle outweighs genetics. 'Genetics are just 20 per cent,' said one. 'Lifestyle choices can change the course of longevity,' said another. The sense of agency is really encouraging.

Instead of decline. many embrace ageing as a journey of wisdom and growth while also admitting they'd like to slow its tougher parts. 'I want to embrace the new me every day,' said one person, 'but I'm also worried about losing mobility.' Acceptance and control, it seems, are a fine balance.

For the under-60s group, ageing well means staying active and independent, looking after mental and physical health, keeping meaningful relationships and living with purpose and peace. Most accept ageing as natural, yet they also believe they have real power to shape how it unfolds. Great! This means most people will be receptive to the seven pillars of pro-ageing regardless of age.

Yes, there are worries about physical decline or loss of independence, but what stands out is the curiosity and self-acceptance that so many voiced. Words like 'wisdom', 'slowing down' and 'living closer to nature' came up repeatedly. This mix of honesty and hope reveals that how we prepare, both inwardly and outwardly, shapes how we experience ageing.

Participants found inspiration for ageing from older friends or relatives, public figures like Dame Helen Mirren and Dame Judi Dench, or by forging their own paths without role models.

Common fears around ageing

As we age, and witness the struggles of our loved ones, it's natural for fear and anxiety around ageing to arise. This comes up time and again both in my own personal surveys and wider research findings on ageing fears. Naming them can help us finally address the elephant in the room, so let's look at a few now:

- **Physical decline** – Both in my research (with the under-60s) and more broadly are concerns about mobility, joint pain, slower healing and menopause-related changes. What's more, a US survey revealed that one in four adults fear losing their physical ability as they age, a concern closely tied to independence and quality of life.
- **Cognitive decline** – The same survey indicated that 15 per cent of respondents feared memory loss, reflecting widespread concern about cognitive decline and conditions like dementia or Alzheimer's that affect memory and daily life. Echoed also in my survey results.
- **Chronic diseases** – Heart disease, hypertension, diabetes, arthritis – all conditions on the rise – raise real concerns about physical limitation and quality of life.
- **Financial insecurity** – Concerns about outliving savings, affording care and maintaining a comfortable lifestyle contribute to anxiety about financial security in later life. Even those aged 29–44 expressed financial anxiety about not having the security their parents had.
- **Loss of independence** – For many elderly, the idea of relying on others for daily tasks, or needing institutional care, feels more frightening than ageing itself.
- **Loneliness and losing loved ones** – Ageing can close in on our circle of friends and family as loved ones depart. Many under-60s feared being 'forgotten' or overlooked, aware that loneliness can seriously affect mental and physical health.
- **Fear of death** – Anxiety about death tends to peak in our 20s and can resurface in our midlife, reflecting the evolving relationship we have with mortality throughout life.

- **Physical appearance** – Wrinkles, weight shifts and grey hair, while natural, can slowly chip away at self-esteem in a culture that prizes youth.

While these fears are real, we don't have to be defined by them. Those in their 60s and older highlight that ageing brings perspective and clarity on what matters most. While anxiety about ageing lives in the mind, its impact is felt in the body.

How ageing shows up in mind and body

The visible signs of ageing are easy to spot – a few lines, greying hair, a slower pace – but the deeper changes often show up as chronic, degenerative conditions. Today, diseases like Alzheimer's, cancer, diabetes, cardiovascular disease and osteoarthritis are on the rise, and the leading causes of death worldwide, driven by inflammation, poor diet, sedentary lifestyles and chronic stress. In other words, our modern lifestyles are accelerating biological ageing and decline.

Each condition reflects a deeper disturbance in our natural *doṣa* balance and digestive strength (***agni***), leading to loss of vitality (*ojas*), and life force (*prāna*) – we'll explore the mechanics further in chapter 3. Osteoarthritis is a degenerative condition, for example; under the *Āyurvedic* lens it reflects dryness in the joints from aggravated ***vāta***, combined with the depletion of bone tissues due to loss of ***kapha*** lubrication in the joints. Diabetes can reflect excess *kapha* resulting in sluggish metabolism and toxin build-up that disrupts sugar metabolism – *see* pp. 37–43 for details on the *doṣas*. When we understand these patterns, our *Āyurvedic* constitution and personal tendencies, we can be more proactive in ageing with awareness instead of reaction.

In *Āyurveda*, we pay equal attention to why something happens (aetiology) and the body's signals of what it is trying to restore (teleology), so we can heal, learn and grow. So, how does the process of ageing begin to express itself?

You may notice your skin beginning to lose its natural glow, moisture and plumpness as the body's nourishment slows down. Your hair may start to thin or turn grey as vitality depletes. The body can feel less grounded, so your joints may feel a little stiffer, muscles a touch weaker, or balance not quite as steady as before. You may find your energy dipping more often and your mind not as sharp as it once was, with moments of forgetfulness, scattered thoughts and sleep that feels lighter than before. You may notice you're more emotionally sensitive and have a tendency towards worry, restlessness or fatigue.

Inside, you may notice your digestion slowing down, reflecting your metabolism is not working quite as efficiently as it once did. You may become prone to heaviness, metabolic toxin build-up (***āma***), and your immune or hormonal balance may feel more sensitive than before. Your breath might not feel as deep, your circulation a little slower and your natural rhythm less in sync with the world around you.

Around menopause, women experience significant physical, emotional and spiritual changes as hormones fluctuate, menstrual cycles pause and rhythms shift. What's often seen as decline is really just the body finding a new balance. Men may notice reduced stamina and reproductive energy marking a transition to a calmer, steadier phase of life.

Ageing is neither a failure nor merely a physical process; it is an invitation to adapt, slow down, simplify and listen more deeply. We already know that prevention is better than a cure but what if we moved the needle even further, towards preserving and protecting our already intelligent, self-healing design?

So, how did ageing start to accelerate faster than it was meant to and what's really behind it?

How modern life drains vitality

How is it possible that two people, both aged 60, can look and feel like they're generations apart? One is vibrant and engaged, the other sluggish and zoned out. What's behind this disparity?

While we appreciate that ageing is a natural process, marked by changes in our tissues, energy and hormones, the pace and experience of it depends on *how* we live. What we eat, how we move, how we think, breathe, sleep, connect with others and our exposure to chronic stress all play a part in the speed of ageing.

At a cellular level, some wear and tear is inevitable. But our environment, habits and mindset can either accelerate or slow our biological clock. Chronic disease and premature ageing have become so common that they seem 'normal' but that does not mean they're *natural*. Just because something is widespread doesn't mean we have to accept it. The body is designed to heal and our system craves regularity and periodic resets.

Āyurveda has long recognised that ageing is shaped by far more than simply a lapse of time: it's the result of many interwoven forces, some beyond our control, like your genome or *prakṛti* (*Āyurvedic* blueprint), which sets the foundation of who you are. But others within our grasp, like your epigenome or ***vikṛti*** (current state of balance/imbalance) reflect how that blueprint is expressed through your lived experience. Everything you're exposed to through food, air, water, sun, chemicals, stress, trauma, culture, relationships etc. forms your exposome – the collection of influences that shape how you age, for better or worse.

In a world that seems to be speeding up, our biology hasn't kept up at the same pace. We live with unprecedented levels of stress, overstimulation from technology, economic and political instability; we're seeing an increase in allergies, intolerances, chronic inflammation, hormonal imbalances and a staggering surge in The Big C (cancer). So, while some factors are written in our genes, much of how we age is shaped through the small, micro habits that either nourish or deplete us. Let's zoom in here.

Habits that age us before our time

Let's face it, modern life isn't designed for vitality. It's fast, noisy, distracting and even if you eat your greens and keep up with your morning yoga, there are distracting habits draining your energy and ageing you long before your time. It's rarely one big event, but a slow build-up of patterns that dim your vitality. Here are some ways this happens knowingly and unknowingly.

The diet trap

Too much sugar doesn't just give you a quick and immediate energy spike, it ages your body from the inside out. When sugar sticks to proteins in your tissues (a process called 'glycation'), skin can look dull, joints stiffen and your metabolism slows down.

Medications like antibiotics, antacids and painkillers can be lifesaving at times, but when overused, they can unsettle the gut's delicate ecosystem. And when the gut is out of sync, so too is everything else, from digestion and immunity to mood and memory.

Layer on to that a diet high in ultra-processed foods (UPFs), pesticide residue and genetically modified ingredients, and it's a perfect storm for inflammation. Tiny toxic particles (like lipopolysaccharides or LPS) can leak from the gut into the bloodstream, triggering a mild but constant immune response that slowly wears the body down. We'll dive deeper into how to create a healthy gut environment in chapter 5 and explore foods that truly nourish in pillar 2.

The lifestyle loopholes

Your body heals while you sleep, but habits like late-night scrolling, bright screens and endless 'to-do' lists rob you of those vital hours. Poor sleep disrupts your hormones and natural detox mechanisms, fogs your mind and depletes your energy. It's one of the most underestimated accelerators of ageing – a lesson I've had to learn the hard way.

Then there's stillness – not the meditative kind, but the couch potato kind. When you don't move enough, your mitochondrial health weakens (she says, as she is glued to the screen as she writes!), slowing your metabolism and draining your energy.

And let's not forget the constant hum of overstimulation: noise, notifications, multitasking. All of this scatters your attention and overstretches your nervous system. Your brain, like your gut, needs quiet time to digest and reset.

The rhythm disruptors

We were meant to rise with the sun, sleep with the stars and sync with the rhythm of the seasons, yet most of us spend our days indoors under artificial light, disconnected from sunlight and nature. When your circadian clock is out of tune, it throws off your hormones, metabolism, sleep and mental clarity. No matter how pristine your diet, your body cannot fully reset if your rhythms are chaotic. This must become a priority in the quest for pro-ageing and is therefore the focus of pillar 1.

The heart of the matter

The greatest youth robber of all? Disconnection. Disconnection from your body, your passions, your purpose, from nature, from community and from your *self*. *Āyurveda* calls this ***tamas*** (inertia), a heavy, dull fog that sets in when you stop feeling inspired, connected or curious.

Toxic relationships, unexpressed emotions, overthinking, chronic fear – all of these contribute to subtle stagnation that weighs down your mind and weakens your body. When you stop feeling fully alive, the body starts to slowly shut down.

Trapped in the trends

Today, health is often packaged as the next revolutionary hack. From juice cleanses, extreme fasting, anti-ageing creams and brain-boosting supplements to synthetic adaptogens, longevity pills, ice baths and sleep trackers, the list is endless. Some have value, but their long-term safety and sustainability are questionable. Most ignore the context of age, gender, stress or *Āyurvedic* constitution (*see* p. 41). True wellness cannot come from outside, happen overnight or need proof before we accept its value. It's an inside job based on how we show up for ourselves.

From disconnection to disease

Not all illness can be avoided, but many imbalances begin long before symptoms appear. *Āyurveda* teaches that time (***kāla***), daily choices and actions (***karma***), misuse of our senses (***ārtha***) and going against our own inner wisdom (***prajñāparādha***) all shape health. When any of these slip out of harmony, imbalance follows and eventually disease finds its way in.

Over time, the sugar, the scrolling, the binge watching, the hustle may seem to bring joy in the moment, but they become habits of depletion and accelerated ageing. The good news? All these vitality thieves are reversible. In part 2, we'll explore simple, timeless practices across the seven pillars of pro-ageing, but for now, let me plant a few seeds with easy swaps to mull over until you reach the juicy part.

Small daily swaps for pro-ageing living

The simple shifts in Table 1.1 below replace habits that drain your vitality with ones that nourish your long-term well-being.

What we need to do less of	What we need to do more of
Over-committing and people-pleasing	Creating space to rest and reset (bookend your days)
Eating on the go, overindulging or skipping meals	Eating consciously while sitting, and at regular times
Ignoring your natural urges (sleep, food, elimination)	Listening to the body's natural needs
Late nights scrolling and midnight munchies	Sleeping early, reading, journalling, connecting with your partner
Overloading the senses	Practising sensory stillness (*pratyāhāra*)
Mindless scrolling, gaming, binge watching	Spending time in nature, nurturing soulful connections and conversations
Eating cold, heavy, processed foods	Eating fresh, seasonal, cooked *sattvic* meals
Multitasking	Being fully engaged with one thing at a time
Comparing, competing, judging, self-criticism	Cultivating contentment and inner joy (*santoṣa*) with what is

Table 1.1 Daily swaps

Age is just a number!

True thing! Science and *Āyurveda* agree that ageing is influenced by how we eat, move, rest and nurture ourselves. With simple, restorative practices - such as meditation, breathwork, plant-based food and connection – we can slow, halt or even reverse biological ageing, preserving youthfulness for longer.

One compelling example is the Counterclockwise study by psychologist Ellen Langer. She found that when elderly men were immersed in an environment that reflected their younger years, complete with the music, décor and conversations of that era, remarkably, they began to show measurable improvements in strength, posture and even vision. Their bodies responded to the shift in perception. The bottom line? Our beliefs about ageing can shape how we age.

One thing is certain: chronological ageing is inescapable – it is simply the number of times we've circled the sun. We can't stop the calendar from turning or the body from moving through life's seasons.

The exciting truth, however, is that we *can* influence our biological age – how our body feels and functions for better or worse. Some people in their 60s radiate vitality, while others in their 30s show signs of premature ageing. The difference lies less in years we've been alive and more in how we care for our body and mind.

In *Āyurveda*, the conversation is entirely different: vitality over vanity. Ageing is seen not as a decline, but as a sacred opportunity – to lean into wisdom, purpose and alignment (*see* chapter 4). While the body may naturally slow down, we can mature without shrinking our spirit. This is *pro-ageing*, a conscious choice to live well, with independence and joy.

Age is an attitude not an impediment

'All that we are is the result of what we have thought.'
The Buddha, Dhammapada 1:1.

Ageing isn't the enemy, fear is! When we stay curious and open, ageing becomes a path of expansion, not decline. Our thoughts, feelings and beliefs about ageing matter: they shape how we live, down to the cellular level. Stories like *I'm too old*, *It's too late* and *What's the point?* gradually chip away at our vitality, while thoughts of love, gratitude and possibility conversely spark healing.

We can instead ask: *What truly matters? Where do I place my energy, my love, my attention, my time?* This shift helps us live with greater presence and intention. Let's pay less attention to (the fear of) death and more intention to honouring life!

Remarkably, we are the only species able to consciously influence our own nervous system – a powerful tool for transformation, don't you think?

Lessons from the super-agers

To close in on the 'vitality gap', it's worth exploring what we can learn from the cultures where long, disease-free and joyful lives are the norm. Dan Buettner's Blue Zones research explored communities like Ikaria (Greece), Okinawa (Japan), Sardinia (Italy), Loma Linda (California, USA) and the Nicoya Peninsula (Costa Rica). In these communities, people consistently live longer, healthier lives, often reaching a centenarian age of 100, not through hacks or treatments, but through simple living. Daily movement in life came naturally through walking, gardening or household chores, rather than confined gym-style exercise. Meals are mostly plant-based, rich in home-grown vegetables, legumes, herbs and healthy fats, eaten mindfully and in moderation. Purpose, what the Okinawans call *ikigai*, infuses each day with meaning, motivating people to rise with joy. Stress melts with rituals such as afternoon naps, quiet reflection, prayer or gathering with loved ones. Elders maintain strong social circles and experience a sense of spiritual belonging, which nurtures emotional resilience. Ageing is not feared; it is respected and embraced. Elders are visible and respected, thriving into their 90s and beyond with grace and strength.

This is what ageing well can – and *should* – look like! *Āyurveda* has always taught us similar lessons: align with nature, honour your rhythms and live with connection and purpose. Pro-ageing is about choosing practices that keep us resilient, joyful and deeply connected. To do this, many of us will need to unlearn old beliefs about ageing and relearn how to approach it with curiosity, openness and respect.

An integrative approach of modern science and *Āyurveda*

Āyurveda has always understood the importance of balance, regeneration and prevention, but it is thanks to contemporary research that these ideas are being validated on a global scale. Advances in imaging, biomarkers, metabolomics, neuroscience, microbiome analysis, genetic research and more have given us a new language to bridge what ancient sages inferred.

Here are just a few examples:

- Modern science is beginning to confirm *Āyurveda*'s understanding on circadian rhythms and chrono-disruption, showing how sleep-wake cycles impact our metabolism, immunity and cognitive function.
- The discovery of epigenetics in the 1940s confirms that lifestyle, diet and mindset can activate or silence genes and affect how long we live.
- Gut health is central to *Āyurveda*, with *agni* (metabolic fire) regarded as vital to immunity, nutrient absorption and vitality – a truth now echoed in modern microbiome and longevity research.

With these tools, we are now perfectly poised to bridge both perspectives, and create a more holistic, intelligent and proactive way to age well.

2

Rasāyana – the art of rejuvenation

'In nature's economy the currency is not money, it is life.'
Vandana Shiva

Before we explore recipes, herbs and practices in part 2, let's first lay the foundations: the philosophy and timeless wisdom that makes *rasāyana* – Āyurveda's treasured branch of rejuvenation for longevity, vitality and immunity – so unique. *Rasāyana* is not just about extending life but about enriching it through every stage of ageing.

In this chapter, we look at:

- How *rasāyana* challenges our modern perceptions of ageing
- How it is defined in the classical texts
- The aims and benefits of *rasāyana*
- How to find your way into *rasāyana* – the two main modes of therapy and its all-encompassing practices
- The importance of cleansing before starting to explore *rasāyana*.

A science that challenges our perceptions

Āyurveda teaches us that while ageing is natural, rapid deterioration is not. Modern research into human longevity suggests that, under the right conditions, we may have the genetic potential to live healthily beyond 100 years.

This is the gift of *rasāyana* – ancient wisdom that offers a shift in perspective towards extending lifespan, enhancing healthspan and closing the 'vitality gap', the disease-free, vibrant years of life. At its core, *rasāyana* is simple: first clear the body of physical and mental *āma*, restore stable digestion, then nourish the tissues (***dhātus***) so they regain strength and resilience.

The real challenge isn't man against time, but our growing disconnection to body, mind, nature, community, breath, purpose, rest and play. Disconnection can lead to burnout, fatigue, insomnia and joint pain, which is now showing up in people barely into their 30s. Many young professionals are already grappling with conditions like diabetes, hypertension and arthritis, health challenges once seen mostly in the elderly. These aren't signs of *old age*, they're signs of imbalance, a loss of rhythm, nourishment and alignment. Sedentary living, erratic eating habits, chronic stress and overuse of synthetic medicines all accelerate premature ageing.

There is no quick fix to closing the 'vitality gap'. Sadly, our default has become one of 'health bypassing', chasing shortcuts, investing in the novelty bio-hacks and getting swept up in the marketing hype of instant wins. *Āyurveda* flips the script by emphasising on practices that align with the body's natural intelligence, clearing what no longer serves and rebuilding what has been worn down – physically, emotionally, energetically and spiritually. It's the long game – from the roots.

What is *rasāyana*?

दीर्घमायुः स्मृतिं मेधामारोग्यं तरुणंवयः।
प्रभावर्णस्वरौदार्यं देहेन्द्रियबलं परम्॥७॥
वाक्सिद्धिं प्रणतिं कान्तिं लभते ना रसायनात्।
लाभोपायो हि शस्तानां रसादीनां रसायनम्॥८॥

dīrgham āyuḥ smṛtiṃ medhām ārogyaṃ taruṇaṃ vayaḥ |
prabhā varṇa svaraudāryaṃ dehendriyabalaṃ param ||
vāksiddhiṃ praṇatiṃ kāntiṃ labhate na rasāyanāt |
lābhopāyo hi śastānāṃ rasādīnāṃ rasāyanam ||

> 'Rasāyana promotes longevity, stable memory and understanding, health and youthfulness. It brings radiance, healthy complexion, a steady voice, composure, strength of the body and senses. It gives reliable speech, the respect of others, and natural attractiveness, through the proper formation of rasa and the succeeding dhātus.'
>
> *Caraka Samhitā*, Cikitsāsthāna. 1.1.7–8

The word *rasāyana* is rich with meaning. *Rasa* refers to the 'vital sap' or essence that sustains all tissues in the body, while *ayana* means 'path'. Together, *rasāyana* is often translated as 'the path of essence' or, in my more poetic interpretation, as 'the art of restoring what keeps us alive, strong and radiant'.

What is profound about *rasāyana* is its holistic effect. The very process that slows ageing and restores youth is the process that builds ***bala*** (resilience and strength) and enhances ***Vyādhi-kṣamatva*** (the body's natural immunity). This highlights that we're not a set of compartmentalised internal systems that needs a pill for every ill, but a complete ecosystem – and *rasāyana* aims to nourish the *whole*.

Rasāyana, therefore, is *Āyurveda*'s all-encompassing branch of *rejuvenation*, working on gut health, immunity, hormones, healthspan and lifespan. It teaches us to eat intelligently using the six *Āyurvedic* tastes (sweet, sour, salty, pungent, bitter and astringent) not just for flavour, but to balance body functions. It can be broken down into the following aspects:

- Diet (***āhāra***) (pillar 2)
- Herbs and formulas (*dravya* and *kalpas*) (pillar 3)
- Behaviour (*ācāra*) (pillars 6 and 7)
- Lifestyle (***vihāra***: movement, rituals, rhythm, therapies) (pillars 1, 2, 4 and 6)
- Mental attitude (***sattva***) (pillar 5)
- Spiritual practice (***ādhyātmika***) (pillar 7)

At a physiological level, *rasa* is the first of the seven *dhātus* (body tissues), as we will learn in chapter 3, and the foundation of physical and mental vitality. When *rasa* is abundant and flowing freely, we feel energised, resilient and mentally clear. When it's weak or obstructed, early signs of imbalance begin to appear.

The World Health Organization defines healthy ageing as 'the process of developing and maintaining the functional ability that enables well-being in older age'. *Rasāyana* aligns perfectly with this vision, with one important distinction – it works best when begun early in life rather than waiting for decline. It calls for us to nourish the body now to help close the 'vitality gap'.

In our current landscape, we're constantly encouraged to 'cut back' with detoxes, restrictive diets and a reductionist approach to health. But for the first time and for the longest of times, *rasāyana* teaches us to replenish, restore and rejuvenate. True health isn't just about what we remove, it's about what we consciously add back in to nourish and rebuild our body for strength and resilience, too.

The aims of *rasāyana*

- To sustain and enhance ***svastha*** over time (*see* p. 36)
- To promote longevity (*āyuṣkara*), vitality (*prāṇa, ojas and tejas*) and spiritual evolution
- To maintain youthfulness *(vaya-sthāpana)*
- To build resilience and strength physically and mentally (*balakara)*
- To enhance the mind (*medhākara)* – intellect, memory, clarity, concentration
- To support our highest potential for a purposeful and fulfilling life.

In practice, *rasāyana* can look like a daily spoonful of ***cyavanaprāśa*** (herbal jam – *see* p. 152), a cup of warm milk with *rasāyana* herbs, the conscious decision to sleep on time or a nourishing meal eaten with presence.

What I *love* most about *rasāyana* is its personalised approach. Whether through food, herbs, movement, breath, behaviour or mindset, it works best when tailored to the individual because like everything in *Āyurveda*, one size does not fit all. It's about the long game – continually tending to your vitality reserves before it runs dry. Working with the guidance of a skilled practitioner can help you fine-tune your journey but the principles and practices in this book are universal, so you can begin exploring *rasāyana* safely and meaningfully on your own.

The benefits of *rasāyana*

Rasāyana is about rebuilding the very foundation of health. When practised consistently, it has the power to:

- Slow down the visible and invisible signs of ageing
- Strengthen immunity and help protect against chronic illness
- Increase daily energy, stamina and clarity
- Support strong digestion and deeper nutrient absorption
- Rebuild tissue health and cellular resilience
- Sharpen memory, focus and cognitive performance
- Calm the nervous system, build resilience to stress and lift mood
- Improve skin radiance and tone from the inside out
- Regulate hormones and sustain overall vitality.

True rejuvenation is not about just adding more years to life, but more life to every year. Consistent self-care can begin to reshape your biology, your energy, mindset and sense of purpose. *Rasāyana* is a return to how we're designed to live and age.

Rasāyana: finding your way in

In order to truly understand *rasāyana*, it helps to understand how it has historically been described and applied, and how that wisdom can be carried over to our modern lives.

Ācārya (sage) **Caraka** describes *rasāyana* in two ways in the *Caraka Saṃhitā – kāmya* and *naimittika. Naimittika is used primarily in cases of disease and its recovery. Kāmya rasāyana* on the other hand focuses on enhancing the quality of life: *prāṇakāmya* for longevity and vitality, *medhakāmya* for enhancement of intellect and memory, and *śrīkāmya* for beauty and radiance. In essence, *rasāyana* supports the body while holding space for consciousness to awaken.

Ācārya Caraka also expressed that *rasāyana* can be delivered via two main *modes* of therapy, giving us a different lens to view *rasāyana*:

1. ***Kuti praveśikā rasāyana*** – a classical *Āyurvedic* seclusion therapy conducted in a purpose-built enclosure to support physical and mental rejuvenation.
2. ***Vātātapika rasāyana*** – a more accessible, everyday *rasāyana* approach integrated into regular life (the focus of this book).

Let's look at both modes of therapy in more detail.

Kuti Praveśikā: the ultimate mind-body reset

The wellness tourism industry is now a booming industry projected to have reached $1.3 trillion by 2025 according to the Global Wellness Institute in their 2022 report. Modern wellness retreats offer a brief curated health break from daily life, though their benefits often fade after returning to routines. But long before modern wellness retreats, there was ***kuti praveśikā*** – a controlled living environment designed to minimise sensory and environmental disturbance and is a part of the ***kāya-kalpa*** rejuvenation process.

Kāya-kalpa, described as 'total body transformation', is a specialised rejuvenation pathway of Āyurveda and Siddha traditions. Its aim was never immortality, but to restore health, slow and even reverse the ageing process, and restore the body's inherent intelligence – a fine art of keeping us youthful while ageing with grace, strength and awareness.

Kuti praveśikā is the most intensive form of *kāya-kalpa*. It literally means 'entering the hut' and that's exactly what happens. A specially designed *kuti* (cottage or chamber) is built in a natural, pollution-free place. After undergoing full purification (like *pañcakarma* – *see* p. 79), the individual enters the hut for 30–120 days, away from light, wind and urbanisation. So, not exactly an escape to a plush wellness resort, but a deeply intentional period of seclusion designed for total renewal of body, mind and spirit.

The environment is carefully controlled with no sudden temperature shifts. The *kuti* traditionally has three concentric chambers, to buffer the outer world. Inside, the person receives nourishment from milk and *rasāyana* formulations and treatments, and remains in meditative stillness. They experience a complete restraint from all worldly distractions and indulgences – physical, social, emotional or sensory. Just calm.

Before entering this type of therapeutic seclusion, many other considerations are factored in. Even the timing of entry is carefully chosen, guided by auspicious astrological alignments.

While there is little outward activity, this is not a passive experience. It requires strong will, discipline and the full support of *Āyurvedic vaidyas* (physicians) and sometimes spiritual guides (brahmins). The goal is more than just rejuvenation, it is to attain a radical rebirth of the physical and mental self. As the ancient texts describe, the person emerges 'as if reborn, with renewed tissues (*dhātus*), softened arteries, a sharp mind, glowing skin, and vibrant energy'.

This intensive *rasāyana* practice was intended for select individuals with the discipline and stability to undertake it – though specialised and rare today, it is still possible to do this process in India. *Ācārya* Caraka and ***Ācārya* Suśruta** would no doubt praise *kuti praveśikā* as the gold standard in 'age-reversal', even referencing the rejuvenation of old and frail *Ācārya* Cyavana, who regained youth after undergoing *rasāyana* therapy in such a setting and later inspired the famed formula now known as *cyavanaprāśa* (*see* pillar 3).

The closest I've come is a 10-day *Vipasannā* silence retreat (a Buddhist meditation practice). And trust me when I say it isn't until we attempt something that truly challenges us that we realise how cluttered our minds and bodies have become. The idea of going inwards can feel immense and what I experienced was not even close to true isolation. How often do you say to yourself, family or friends, 'Oh I really need a holiday/break'? The question is – a holiday or break from what exactly?

Few of us can endure a forest *kuti* for 90 days of silence and seclusion. Yet the principle remains – healing happens when we pause, cleanse, nourish and align. Silence, solitude and simplicity are the true luxuries for our overfed, overstimulated yet undernourished lives.

Vātātapika rasāyana: everyday rejuvenation for real life

Most of us have families, jobs and responsibilities, which is exactly why *Ācārya* Caraka and *Ācārya* Vagbhaṭa explicitly encourage the *vātātapika* path. Unlike *kuti praveśikā*, which calls for isolation and strict discipline, *vātātapika* invites us to integrate *rasāyana* into our daily life – phew!

Designed for the householder, *rasāyana* can work by steadily integrating foods and practices with intention and proper guidance in a real-life setting. This approach simply calls for consistency. That may look like:

- Taking *rasāyana* herbs suited to your constitution
- Adjusting your diet to be more *sattvic* (pure, nourishing)
- Strengthening your daily rhythms, sleep, mealtimes and mental focus
- Minimising stimulation and emotional triggers
- Choosing rejuvenative rituals that you can stick to.

While it may not bring the same rapid transformation as *kuti praveśikā*, the cumulative effect of daily *rasāyana* practices is still profound, boosting energy, strength (*bala*), supporting immunity (*ojas*) and preserving clarity and strength well into our maturation phase.

To integrate *rasāyana* is to restore what's depleted, strengthen what's weak and bring balance where there's excess – this is the science of rejuvenation! Imagine waking up each morning with the same spark you had as a child, rising with energy, clarity and excitement. This is the promise of *rasāyana* when you focus on your future self as much as your present self.

Think of *vātātapika* as your daily deposit into a long-term vitality account. Small actions, done consistently, yield powerful results over time. And that, for most of us, is the real magic.

You can't nourish an overloaded body!

There is a time and a process for everything. You wouldn't paint over a wall covered in dust or grime and expect it to look fresh and new. You'd clean it first, fix the cracks and prepare the surface so that the new paint sticks and looks flawless. Nobody wants cowboys doing their decorating! Your body works the same way. Before it can absorb nourishment through food, herbs, rest or even love, your *agni* (metabolic fire), natural detox organs (like the liver, kidneys and gut) need to be functioning well. Otherwise, you're just layering wellness on top of waste – we explore this further in chapter 5.

In *Āyurveda*, when *āma* (undigested metabolic residue) is present, deep internal cleansing must always come first. It clears the channels, rekindles metabolic fire (*agni*) and lays the foundation for true rejuvenation (*rasāyana*). Without it, no superfood, tonic or therapy can be fully received by the body, despite the potential health benefits. It would be like scattering seeds over weeds in hope of a harvest.

The challenge today? Detox has become a trend. 'I'm on a detox' usually means a few green juices or skipping wine for a week or missing a few meals. And while these may bring short-term results, they rarely go deep enough. The truth is that many people are living in a constant state of low-level toxicity. These include both *endogenous* toxins (*āma*, produced within the body due to poor digestion and metabolism) and *exogenous* toxins (*āgantu*) absorbed from pollution, synthetic chemicals, stress and overstimulation.

Even thoughts can be toxic. The ancient *siddhas,* **yogic** alchemists of the Tamil region, spoke of mental āma, the residue from unprocessed emotions, chronic overthinking or living out of alignment with one's nature. This blocks energy flow just as much as a clogged gut or sluggish liver. So how do we truly reset? Well, we will dive into this through the seven pillars.

It helps to think of *rasāyana* as a process, not a pill. A living, breathing system that unfolds in stages, each one preparing the body for the next: cleanse first, then rejuvenate. A simple way to think of it is:

Get clean → Stay clean → Try not to get overloaded → Then *rasāyana*

- **Get clean**: When necessary, through deep purification practices like *pañcakarma*, periodic fasting (***upavāsa***), lightening practices (***laṅghana***), and supportive herbal therapies. This clears *āma* (toxins), rekindles metabolic fire (*agni*) and resets the system at a functional level. Think of it as deep spring-cleaning for your inner world.
- **Stay clean**: With daily and seasonal routines (***dinacaryā*** and ***ṛtucaryā***), mindful eating, *agni*-aligned meal timings or light fasting where appropriate. This is the regular housekeeping that keeps your *agni* stable, and body and mind clear.
- **Try not to get overloaded again**: Respect your digestive intelligence. Avoid eating when you're not hungry, emotional,

rushed or full. It's time to refrain from the junk food, junk thoughts, social overload and overstimulation. Ask yourself: *Does it nourish me?*

- **Then . . . *rasāyana***: Once the system is clear and steady, the body can rebuild and rejuvenate. This is where tissues (*dhātus*) rebuild, *ojas* (vitality) and *tejas* (radiance) strengthen and *prāṇa* (life force) flows freely. It's where the magic of pro-ageing begins and is the missing piece in most longevity conversations today.

We're often so fixated on what we should cut out in our quest to feel 'clean and healthy' that we don't realise that true well-being is equally about what we put back in – the nourishment, the joy, the rest and resilience. Detox may clear the vessel but *rasāyana* fills the cup.

My observation as a practitioner for 20+ years, has been that many seekers come to *Āyurveda* with the goal of purification through its esteemed cleansing, fasting and *pañcakarma* processes. Contrary to popular belief, health isn't found by staying in a constant cleanse mode. In the classical approach, cleansing is just the preparation – a functional reset so that the body can receive nourishment to support our eco system both for our present and future self. The real health goal for pro-ageing is to preserve life by building strong and stable tissues and sustainable vitality (*ojas*). What I often see now is plenty of cleansing and very little rebuilding. Over time this becomes depleting and particularly *vāta*-aggravating in a maturing body.

Well-being becomes more meaningful when we understand what's unfolding within the body, so next, we turn to the *Āyurvedic* anatomy of ageing to help us understand *rasāyana* in more context.

3

Āyurvedic anatomy of ageing (eight key concepts)

'If you begin to understand what you are without trying to change it, then what you are undergoes a transformation.'

Jiddu Krishnamurti

In *Āyurveda*, timely, natural ageing (*kālaja jarā*) is a gentle and gradual process. Premature ageing (*akālaja jarā*) occurs when signs and symptoms of ageing show up too soon, often due to chronic stress, erratic routines, poor nourishment and a disconnection to nature. *Āyurveda* teaches us that premature ageing is neither inevitable nor irreversible.

Rasāyana (rejuvenation) opens a more nuanced picture of biological ageing; one guided by rhythms, elements and energies that can be nourished and supported. This chapter explores the *Āyurvedic* landscape of the inner systems, flows and subtle forces that shape how the mind and body age. When you understand the terrain, you can navigate it wisely and begin to see how the magic of *rasāyana* comes to life.

In this chapter we break down:

- The *Āyurvedic* definition of health – what it truly means to be *svastha*, or 'established in the Self'
- Eight key *Āyurvedic* concepts for health and ageing:
  1. The three *doṣas* – the governing forces of body and mind that influence how we age
  2. *Agni* and *āma* (metabolic fire and toxins) – the twin roots of ageing and rejuvenation
  3. ***Sapta dhātus*** (seven sustaining body tissues) – the process that nourishes our tissues and sustains vitality

4. *Subtle energies: prāṇa, tejas, ojas* – the subtle trio that powers resilience and vitality
5. *Srotas* (body channels) – the internal pathways of circulation, communication and flow
6. The ***manas*** (mind) – understanding how perception, emotion and awareness evolve with the body
7. *Kāla* (time) – the natural sculptor of our cycles, seasons and ageing process
8. Western mechanisms and the *Āyurvedic* mirror – bridging ancient wisdom and modern science.

What is a healthy life?

No matter which health system I explore, nothing comes close to the depth and completeness of *Āyurveda's* definition of health. To embrace the *rasāyana* approaches in this book, it helps to understand what a healthy life actually is.

While we readily accept health as merely the absence of disease, *Āyurveda* asks us to look deeper by offering a complete system of preventative well-being, one that is inherently pro-ageing, supporting longevity *and* vitality.

Health (***svasthya***) in *Āyurveda* is a state of dynamic alignment of mind, body and soul. You recognise it when you feel nourished yet light in the body, clear in the mind and senses, and deeply aligned and rooted in yourself. Or to put it another way, it is when our digestion, sleep, energy, mind, emotions and spiritual connection function in harmony.

Let's break it down:

समदोषः समाग्निश्च समधातु-मलक्रियः ।
प्रसन्नात्मेन्द्रियमनाḥ स्वस्थ इत्यभिधीयते ॥

samadoṣaḥ samāgniś ca samadhātu-malakriyaḥ |
prasannātmendriya-manāḥ svastha iti abhidhīyate ||

Suśruta Saṁhitā, Sūtrasthāna. 15.41

This poignant definition of health translates that a person is only considered truly healthy when:

- The *doṣas* (bio-energetic forces: *vāta*, ***pittā***, *kapha*) are balanced according to your constitution
- The *agni* (digestive and metabolic fires) function optimally
- The *dhātus* (body tissues) are well nourished
- The ***malas*** (waste elimination) are well-functioning
- The ***indriyas*** (senses) are clear and sharp
- The *manas* (mind) is in a state of calm harmony
- The *ātman* (soul) is content and at peace.

The aim of *Āyurveda* is to attain *svastha* - 'to be established in the self', where we are in a state of complete balance in the functional health of the body, mind and spirit. The aim of *rasāyana* subsequently is to sustain good *svastha* over the course of your life, but to also build on this foundation.

Embracing *svasthavṛtta*

To achieve *svastha*, Āyurveda gives guidance on healthy living - ***svasthavṛtta*** - to maintain health and prevent diseases. It emphasises daily and seasonal routines (*dinacaryā* and ***ṛtucaryā***), diet (*āhāra*), lifestyle (*vihāra*), ethical conduct (***sadvṛtta***), mental hygiene (***satvavajaya***) and spiritual well-being (*ādhyātmika*). Through the seven pillars in part 2, we will explore the practical ways to slow down and even prevent premature ageing or age-related conditions but before we do, let's get into the nuts and bolts of *Āyurveda's* anatomy of ageing.

So, what truly drives the ageing process from an *Āyurvedic* perspective?

As time passes, the body's inner balance begins to shift: *vāta doṣa* gradually increases, the *dhātus* (tissues) begin to deplete, *āma* (waste) can accumulate, and the vital forces that sustain life - *ojas, prāṇa* and *agni* - gently decline. Alongside these natural physical changes, our sense of connection, purpose and inner clarity can waver - threads we'll explore more deeply in the next chapter.

Eight key *Āyurvedic* concepts for health and ageing

To understand how *Āyurveda* guides graceful ageing, we turn to eight foundational concepts that form the scaffolding for protecting health and vitality. Each concept builds on the definition of *svastha*, deepening our understanding of how the body is nourished, how it depletes, and how ageing unfolds. Together, they prepare us to explore the practicalities of *rasāyana*.

Āyurvedic concept 1: the three *doṣas*

In *Āyurveda*, the *doṣas* are the three guiding bio-energies that shape how we look, feel, think and behave throughout life. Though they may seem abstract, they are living forces that give us motion, transformation and structure. They arise from the five great elements (***pañca mahābhūtas***). The three *doṣas* are:

1. *Vāta* (air and space) - directs movement and communication
2. *Pittā* (fire and water) - drives transformation and metabolism
3. *Kapha* (water and earth) - provides structure and stability.

Together they create an energetic blueprint for all your physiological and psychological processes; they are the dynamic trio that determine growth, transformation and decay. Each one of us is born with a unique blend of these bio-energetic forces, known as *prakṛti* (your constitution). For most of us, one or two *doṣas* usually take the lead, shaping our strengths, personality, tendencies and vulnerabilities.

Your current *doṣhic* state (*vikṛti*) reflects imbalances shaped by diet, lifestyle, stress, emotions, seasons, time and environment. I always think of *prakṛti* as our 'nature' and *vikṛti* as our 'nurture' - and they both influence how each of us will age.

When the *doṣas* are balanced, the body's natural intelligence works smoothly - digestion and energy remain steady, and vitality is sustained. When they fall out of balance, our inner harmony falters, leading to fatigue, inflammation and premature ageing.

Each *doṣa* has distinct characteristics, qualities and plays specific roles in the body and mind. The table below gives you a quick overview for reference:

	Vāta	*Pittā*	*Kapha*
Function in body and mind	Movement, communication, physical and mental activity, creativity and adaptability	Digestion, metabolism, transformation, comprehension, emotions, vision	Lubrication, structure, stability, cohesion, endurance
Qualities	Cold, light, dry, irregular, rough, quick, mobile, changeable, subtle	Hot, light, dry, penetrating, oily, sharp, intense, acidic	Heavy, slow, steady, cool, soft, oily, solid, dense, moist, dull
Typical traits	Thin frame, quick speech, active/ creative mind, dry skin, bursts of energy followed by slumps, light sleep, sensitive digestion, excitable, imaginative	Medium build, warm body, sharp intellect, fair complexion, strong digestion, clear focus, confident, assertive, energetic, lustrous skin	Large frame, strong build, calm and loving nature, steady, loyal, thick hair, radiant eyes, preference for sweet tastes, regular digestion
Expression of Imbalance	Weight loss, constipation, dry skin, worry and anxiety, insomnia, easily stressed, joint pain or arthritis, bloating, restlessness	Irritability, short temper, argumentative, inflammation, acid reflux or heartburn, indigestion, ulcers and skin rashes, intolerant to heat	Weight gain, fluid retention, sluggish digestion, respiratory issues (asthma, congestion), depression, attachment, greed

Table 3.1 Properties of each *doṣa*

Knowing your *prakṛti/vikṛti* helps you understand yourself better and tailor the *rasāyana* approaches in this book to your true nature. Do you resonate with one or two of the *doṣas* in the table? If so, it may be an indicator of the dominant *doṣa in your prakṛti*. If you'd like to explore your unique constitution more deeply, my first book, *Ayurveda: Ancient Wisdom for Modern Wellbeing,* is a good place to start, or you can work with an *Āyurvedic* practitioner for personalised *rasāyana* guidance (*see* Resources, pp. 271–2).

True 'balance' means living in a way that minimises your *vikṛti* and aligns with your *prakṛti* – your personalised state of equilibrium. Over time, though, no matter your constitution, we all gradually move into the *vāta* stage of life.

As the force of movement and change, *vāta*'s qualities become more noticeable: dryness of the skin and hair, wrinkles, prominent veins, lighter sleep and irregular digestion. There may be a reduction in immunity, hormone production, sweating and muscle mass. Mentally, the rise of *vāta* may manifest as scattered focus, worry or anxiety. If *vāta* is already dominant in your *prakṛti*, these signs may show up louder and/or sooner.

Pittā-dominant folks may see premature greying, hair thinning or sensitivity in the skin. *Kapha*-dominant individuals may notice slower metabolism and easier weight gain. These fluctuations explain why ageing looks and feels different for everyone. Below, we take a deeper look at how each *doṣa* expresses itself when it's both in balance and in an imbalanced state, and actions we can take:

1. ***Vāta* – the energy of movement**

   Vāta is light, cool, mobile and dry in nature and is the energy of movement in the body and mind from breath and blood flow to nerve signals and communication.

   When balanced, people with *vāta* dominance are slim-built, alert, enthusiastic, adaptable and creative. But when life gets hectic or overstimulating – maybe due to irregular mealtimes, sleep or travel, *vāta* can tip out of balance. Often leading to an increase in dryness, fear, anxiety, restlessness, scattered focus and trouble sleeping.

   To balance *vāta*, regular routines and rituals that are simple, grounding, warming and oil-based are the best antidotes to restore balance.

2. ***Pittā* – the energy of transformation**
   Pittā's nature is fiery, sharp and intense and its primary role is digestion, metabolism and the transformation of everything from food to sensory inputs and thoughts.

   When balanced, people with *pittā* dominance have a medium build with a strong appetite, radiant skin and are driven by purpose. However, excess stress, competition, spicy food and intense heat can overheat *pittā*. This can trigger irritability, anger, inflammation, skin irritation and tendencies towards self-criticism or perfectionism.

   The best way to cool off and maintain vibrancy without burning out is time in nature, cooling foods, adequate rest, laughter and compassion.
3. ***Kapha* – the energy of stability**
   Described as heavy, cold, slow and steady, *kapha* provides structure, stability and softness to the body and mind.

   When balanced, people with *kapha* dominance have a robust build, a calm and warm disposition, bags of empathy and are overall, the most resilient. But when *kapha* rises due to inactivity, emotional inertia or overeating, there will be a tendency to lethargy, congestion, weight gain or holding on to possessions, relationships and routines that don't serve.

   Incorporating movement, lightness, inspiration and variety is essential to keep *kapha* flowing so it doesn't become stuck and stagnant.

Doṣas and the stages of life

Āyurveda teaches that life itself moves in rhythm with the *doṣas*, influencing how we grow and mature. Each phase carries its own intelligence: *kapha* builds, *pittā* transforms and *vāta* liberates. When we respect these tides, ageing becomes more of a deepening than a decline.

Let's examine each phase of life in turn now:

1. **The spring of life – *kapha* (0–18 years)**
   Our early years when *kapha* dominates are a time of rapid growth, building tissue and forming resilience and vitality for later life.

Instinctively, children crave sweet, grounding foods to support growth. Likewise, the young mind is like a sponge for everything and thrives when there is a feeling of safety, stability and love. The best support for this season is routines, warm, nourishing foods, light spices and plenty of active playtime.

2. **The summer of life - *pittā* (18–55 years)**
   Our adulthood is dominated by *pittā* and it's a time to be immersed in digesting and metabolising life through productivity and purpose. A natural time for developing talents, knowledge, skills and achieving goals while nurturing relationships, family life and passions.

   During this time, there can be a tendency to push too hard, which can result in exhaustion and burnout. Our best allies during this season are grounding meals, purposeful pauses and regular self-care.
3. **The autumn and winter of life - *vāta* (55+ years)**
   Our mature years are dominated by the lightness and sensitivity of *vāta* and with it come the space for wisdom, reflection, creativity and spiritual deepening. During this time digestion slows, sleep becomes lighter, skin becomes drier and the nervous system feels more delicate.

   These years call for more warmth and grounding. Favouring warmth, routine, moist, nourishing meals, gentle movement, creative pursuits, deep rest and social and spiritual connection are some of the best ways we can support this stage.

Āyurvedic concept 2: *agni* and *āma* – metabolic fire and toxins

In *Āyurveda*, balancing the *doṣas* and maintaining a healthy gut go hand in hand. At the core of this balance are your *agnis* (metabolic fires), which govern how you break down, absorb and eliminate what you eat. If you have a balanced digestion (***samāgni***), you're already winning. When your digestive fire is steady, you absorb nutrients well, build resilience and feel light, energised and clear. Balanced *agni* supports healthy appetite, easy elimination, radiant skin and a steady mood. When it becomes disturbed, *āma* (undigested metabolic residue) builds up and that's where trouble begins.

Our digestive fire can go off balance in three ways, each reflecting the qualities of one of the *doṣas*.

1. ***Viṣamāgni*** (*vāta*) is an irregular digestion with a tendency towards bloating, gas and variable hunger.
2. ***Tikṣṇāgni*** (*pittā*) is a sharp digestion and prone to acidity, intense hunger and irritability.
3. ***Mandāgni*** (*kapha*) is a slow and sluggish digestion, causing heaviness, low appetite and weight gain.

When digestion is too fast, too slow or just confused, even wholesome food can turn into *āma* (a heavy, sticky metabolic residue formed from incomplete digestion and processing) that clogs your system and dims your vitality. Add in stress, cold or processed foods, overeating or emotional turmoil, and you've got the perfect storm for digestive disruption. Over time, as *āma* accumulates, it can show up as inflammation, fatigue, brain fog and weakened immunity, giving rise to many health conditions.

Āyurveda gives us simple but powerful rituals to keep *agni* strong (*see* chapter 5). We're talking about warm, home-cooked meals, regular mealtimes, no mindless snacking, and sipping warm water. It's not just *what* you eat, but *how* you eat that makes all the difference. Move your body, manage stress and rest well. Your gut will thank you. For more on personalising your approach, you'll find deeper guidance in my book, *Ayurveda: Ancient Wisdom for Modern Wellbeing*.

How your body gets nourished

Nourishment isn't just about what you eat for your daily energy, but how deeply what you consume literally becomes you (including food, water, breath, impressions).

Our bodies are wildly intelligent. With each meal, they break down and absorb what's useful and release what's not. Digestion may only take three to six hours, but the full conversion of food from a single meal into the seven body tissues can take 30 to 40 days.

Āyurveda describes this through two linked processes: the three stages of digestion, and nourishment of the *sapta dhātus* (seven sustaining body tissues). Let's walk through each step:

Three stages of digestion

Āyurveda sees digestion as a living, intuitive process, led in turn by each of the three *doṣas*:

1. Phase 1: Mouth to upper stomach (*kapha* stage) – Digestion begins the moment food touches your tongue. This is the *kapha* stage, where chewing and saliva begin to break down and moisten the food, sending cues to the stomach to get ready.
2. Phase 2: Stomach and small intestines (*pittā* stage) – Here the digestive fire (***jaṭharāgni*** – referred as *agni* throughout this book) in the stomach takes charge, supported by the liver and pancreas. The food is transformed into a nutrient-rich liquid called ***āhāra rasa*** (akin to chyme, a semi-liquid mixture of partially digested food).

   In the small intestines, *āhāra rasa* meets the five elemental fires (***bhūtāgnis***), which refine the substance into elemental components space, air, fire, water and earth – preparing the nutritional fluid that will nourish the *sapta dhātus*.
3. Phase 3: colon (*vāta* stage) – The final stage of digestion takes place in the colon, where waste is formed and is ready for elimination.

When these three phases flow with ease, digestion is complete, nourishment is absorbed, waste is cleared and the body stays free of *āma*. A steady fire becomes the foundation for *rasāyana* foods and herbs to fully nourish the body tissues that follow.

Āyurvedic concept 3: *sapta dhātus* – nourishment of the seven body tissues

Now that we've understood how food is broken down, let's look at how it becomes you. The body's seven sustaining tissues (*sapta dhātus*) are nourished through a beautiful sequential process known as ***dhātu parināma*** (*see* Figure 3.1, overleaf).

In simple terms, each *dhātu* is nourished in turn. The first, *rasa* (plasma) feeds the second, ***rakta*** (blood), which nourishes ***māṃsa*** (muscle), and so on, all the way to ***śukra/ārtava*** (reproductive tissue) – the most refined tissue that gives rise to *ojas* (the nectar of vitality).

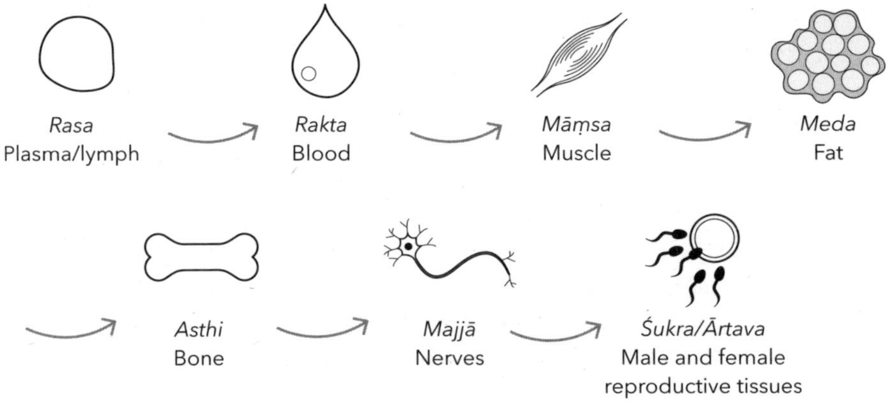

Figure 3.1 The body's seven tissues, the *sapta dhātus*

When this process functions efficiently, we maintain well-formed tissues and call it ***dhātusāmya***.

The quality of nourishment moving through the seven tissues depends on the strength of the metabolic 'fire' of each tissue (***dhātvagni***). When the tissue fire burns steadily, each *dhātu* absorbs what it needs to sustain itself and passes the refined nourishment along. But if any of the fires are weak, tissues can become depleted (loss of strength, tone or density) or congested (as in excess fat or fluid retention).

If the digestive process is poor from the start, *āma* can also enter the nutrient stream and affect the process. This can disrupt tissue function and weaken immunity, giving rise to disease and accelerated ageing – the deeper truth behind the saying: 'You are what you do *and* don't digest'.

How your tissues get depleted

As we age, our body's ability to transform food into strong, resilient tissues becomes more delicate. *Agni* begins to dim, and the light, dry and mobile qualities of *vāta doṣa* naturally rise. If this is not addressed it can slowly diminish tissue integrity and weaken *dhātvagni*, leading to gradual depletion and – you guessed it – ageing!

Āyurvedic concept 4: the subtle energies: *prāṇa, tejas* and *ojas*

Each *doṣa*, when in balance, gives rise to its own subtle essence: *vāta* flows into *prāṇa*, *pittā* radiates as *tejas*, and *kapha* becomes *ojas*. While the *doṣas* govern the physical body and its functions, these refined expressions, sometimes called the *sukshma doṣas* (subtle energies) belong to the subtle body. Together they form the foundation of *vitality* – a word you'll see often in this book. When we speak of *vitality*, we're referring to the optimal essence of this trio that powers your body and mind to heal and flourish. They sustain everything from energy and clarity to resilience and longevity. When *prāṇa*, *tejas* and *ojas* are optimal, we thrive: physically, mentally and emotionally – the very essence of health (*svasthya*).

As we age, nurturing and optimising these subtle energies becomes essential for longevity and vitality, and is the aim of *rasāyana*. I like to think of them as the currency for pro-ageing, an inner wealth you will learn to strengthen through the tools, techniques and rituals shared in part 2. Let's understand each one here:

- ***Ojas*** – The subtle essence of *kapha*, *ojas is* your body's inner reservoir of strength, immunity and endurance. It's built slowly from the nourishment we absorb, through food, rest, thoughts, emotions and lived experience. As the foundation of tissue health and resilience, *ojas is* what helps us bounce back, heal deeply and stay well in the face of stress or illness.

  Strong *ojas is* key to both healthspan and lifespan, supporting regeneration, stability, strength (*bala*) and radiance. Low *ojas* shows up as fatigue, anxiety, fragility or depletion. Self-massage, milk-based tonics and good sleep are just a few examples of *rasāyana* practices that build *ojas*.
- ***Prāṇa*** – *Prāṇa*, the subtle essence of *vāta*, is the vital life force that fuels breath, movement and mental activity. It governs all flow in the body and mind, from the rhythm of your inhale to the spark of your thoughts. Flowing through the ***nādīs*** (subtle energy channels) of the subtle body, *prāṇa* is the animating force that connects your inner and outer worlds. When *prāṇa* flows freely, you feel alert, inspired and deeply alive.

Prāṇa sustains mental clarity, emotional steadiness and cellular intelligence. When it's depleted, vitality fades and we feel flat, exhausted and just a little lifeless. As the living bridge between the body and consciousness, *prāṇa* is quite literally the difference between life and death. Tending to it is the key to graceful ageing. Unlike the stored energy (*ojas*), *prāṇa* must be continually replenished through conscious breathing, movement, time in nature, rest and vibrant, living foods (*see* pillar 5).

- ***Tejas*** – The subtle essence of *pittā*, *tejas* is your inner light, the radiance that gives lustre to your eyes, glow to your skin and clarity to your mind. It governs transformation on every level, helping you metabolise at the subtle level: not just food, but thoughts, emotions and life's experiences. When *tejas* is balanced it fuels clarity, intelligence and sharp communication between body and mind.

  As we age, steady *tejas* helps prevent burnout, mental fog and dullness. Gentle practices like meditation, restful pauses and a diet that supports your digestive fire can help maintain your inner spark and keep your intellect bright.

Protecting *ojas* through *brahmacharya*

One of the most effective ways to protect *ojas*, the body's essence of vitality and immunity, is ***brahmacharya***. Beyond its traditional meaning of celibacy, it refers to consciously channelling sexual energy and mental desires so that *śukra* (reproductive tissue) is not wasted through excess stimulation or indulgence. By practising moderation and mindful restraint, *brahmacharya* becomes a subtle form of *rasāyana* – supporting resilience and vitality. Indian spiritual teacher Swami Sivananda Saraswati called brahmacharya 'the master key' to health and longevity.

Vitality check-in

How do you currently weigh in on the vitality scale? Reflect on each of the following questions and answer them honestly. Notice which already feels strong and support your *ojas*, *prāna* and *tejas*, and where your energy might need gentle attention to enhance nourishment, balance and clarity.

1. **Nourishment and grounding (*ojas*)**
   - ☐ I eat freshly prepared, wholesome meals that leave me feeling nourished and satisfied.
   - ☐ I maintain regular mealtimes and avoid skipping meals or overeating.
   - ☐ I get sufficient, restful sleep and usually wake up feeling refreshed and ready for the day.
   - ☐ I rarely fall ill and recover quickly from illness if I do.
   - ☐ I take time to restore myself through self-care, such as body massage, nature walks or moments of stillness.
2. **Radiance and clarity (*tejas*)**
   - ☐ I feel mentally clear, focused and able to concentrate without frequent distraction.
   - ☐ I engage in activities that stimulate me intellectually and creatively, such as reading, learning or problem-solving.
   - ☐ I express my thoughts and emotions clearly, confidently and honestly.
   - ☐ I feel inspired and passionate about what I do, whether it's for work, family or fun.
   - ☐ I spend time in natural light or sunlight and feel energised by it.
3. **Energy and flow (*prāṇa*)**
   - ☐ I consciously connect with my breath daily, especially in moments of stress or fatigue.
   - ☐ I spend time in nature to recharge my energy, such as sitting by a river or gardening.
   - ☐ I cultivate positive relationships and spend time with people who uplift and inspire me.
   - ☐ I practise gentle movement, yoga or ***prāṇāyāma*** to support my energy.
   - ☐ I allow time for rest, relaxation, meditation or prayer to restore inner stillness and balance.

As we progress through part 2 of this book you will gain wisdom, tools and techniques that will enhance all three subtle energies – you can revisit this checklist to monitor your development.

Āyurveda's je ne sais quoi

I remember studying *ojas* (vital essence) for the first time nearly 25 years ago and being fascinated to learn there are two kinds. The *ojas* I refer to in this book is *apara ojas*, the essence that circulates through the body, nourishing the tissues and supporting immunity, strength and vitality. But there is also *para ojas, the* supreme *ojas*, located in the heart with a fixed quantity of eight drops (*aṣṭa-bindu*). While *apara ojas* slowly diminishes as we age, *para ojas is* present from conception *and* remains constant until the end of our life and is irreplaceable. It is the seat of life, sustaining consciousness and vitality at the deepest level. I hold this concept sacredly, as if *para ojas* were a personal treasure chest of our *inner elixir* - not literally measurable drops, but symbolic of the finite spark of life we all carry within.

Āyurvedic concept 5: *srotas* – keeping your inner pathways clear

Your body functions through an intricate network of channels known in *Āyurveda* as ***srotas***. These are pathways through which nourishment, breath, waste and energy flow through your body. We can easily observe the physical channels, like the respiratory, urinary and digestive, but we also have more subtle energetic pathways called *nādīs* through which *prāṇa* flows, influencing nerve signals, thoughts and emotions. The subtle channels work through the deeper ***kośas*** (our energetic and mental sheaths), which we explore further in chapter 4.

According to *Āyurveda,* longevity and vitality depend on keeping these channels open and clear. On a physical level, nutrients reach your tissues and toxins are easily cleared; on an energetic level, *prāṇa* and emotions flow with ease. But as we age or experience stress, struggle with poor digestion or accumulation of *āma*, these pathways can become blocked. This may show up as constipation, sluggish circulation or mental fog.

Practices like cleansing therapies, conscious movement, steady digestion and living in harmony with your constitution all help keep *srotas* clear so that you can benefit from *rasāyana* nourishment at every layer of your being.

Āyurvedic concept 6: *manas* – the power of the mind

In *Āyurveda*, *manas* (the mind) acts as a bridge between the body and soul, constantly processing and interpreting information received through our senses by the intellect, and subsequently navigating our decisions and actions. The mind shapes how we perceive health, ageing and life itself. As we age, we want to enhance the quality of *sattva* (clarity, calm, wisdom), so we can live with peace, resilience and insight.

When our mind is overstimulated, the quality of ***rajas*** (restlessness) can cloud our clarity; if we lack engagement, the quality of *tamas* (inertia) can drain our motivation. Either way, mental clarity and emotional steadiness decline, disturbing the subtle energy of *prāṇa*. Without a steady mind, we lose the sense of connection to ourselves, others and something greater, resulting in a lack of joy and meaning, subtly accelerating ageing.

When our *manas* is calm and clear, we absorb the benefits of *rasāyana* at every layer of our being. In pillars 5, 6 and 7 we'll explore *rasāyana* practices to sustain mental balance, nourish *prāṇa* and deepen meaningful connections – keeping you on a pro-ageing trajectory.

Āyurvedic concept 7: *kāla* – time, our deepest teacher

In Vedic wisdom, *kāla* (time) is more than ticking clocks: it is a living force. Time does not move linearly but in cycles, often described as the *kāla chakra*, or the wheel of time. The choices and actions of the past, known as *karma*, ripple into the present, shaping how we live and what we experience. Our choices and actions today sow the seeds of tomorrow.

Sometimes it can feel like time is slipping away, like there's never *enough* of it. Be honest: how often do you say 'I don't have time' or 'I'm too busy'? Perhaps the question is – what are we choosing to *make time* for?

Like money, time can be wasted (dead time), spent (for quick returns) or invested (soulful returns) – the kind that nourishes longevity and *rasāyana* living. Time is our greatest flex! It is the only resource that is finite. We all get the same 24 hours in a day, but how we use them defines the texture of our days and shapes our experience.

The Vedas (India's oldest sacred texts) invite us to look at time differently – not as something to chase or control, but as a sacred container that we live *within*. What if time wasn't something you lost, but something you honoured? Honouring time means embracing it as a rhythm that flows through nature, through your body and through the seasons of your life. Some moments are made for action, others for rest, connection or reflection. When you stop chasing time and start living *with* it, everything softens – we can truly be here now. Ironically, it took me some 'time' to be at peace with this reality!

I've found that stepping away from the digital buzz, even briefly, opens space for what really matters: soulful conversations, stillness, laughter, time in nature. It's not about having more time; it's about being in an aligned relationship with it. So much of life begins to shift when we are mindful of what we say yes to.

Pro-ageing exercise: how do you relate to time?

This simple exercise helps you notice whether your mindset leans towards what I like to call a time-anxious (rushing against time) or a time-aligned (flowing with time) pattern, so you can see where shifts may bring more ease and balance. Tick each of the following statements that resonate with you (be sincere).

Part 1

- ☐ I often feel like there just aren't enough hours in the day.
- ☐ I feel overwhelmed by constant digital notifications and messages.
- ☐ My work or responsibilities often spill over into my personal time.
- ☐ Sometimes I stay up late worrying about unfinished tasks.
- ☐ I frequently feel pressured to meet deadlines or keep up with others.
- ☐ I find it hard to relax, even when I have free time.
- ☐ I feel guilty when I take time for myself.
- ☐ Often I multitask to get things done faster.

→

- ☐ I worry that I'm not making enough progress towards my goals.
- ☐ I find it difficult to disconnect from work or social media.
- ☐ Sometimes I sacrifice sleep or self-care to keep up with my obligations.
- ☐ I prefer structured routines and planning over spontaneous activities.

Score: _______

Part 2

- ☐ Often I lose track of time when I'm absorbed in something I enjoy.
- ☐ I can easily disconnect from social media and digital distractions.
- ☐ I feel at peace with who I am, regardless of external achievements.
- ☐ I value taking time to reflect and recharge.
- ☐ I am comfortable spending time alone and enjoy my own company.
- ☐ I prioritise experiences and personal growth over material success.
- ☐ I feel connected to something greater than myself (nature, community, spirituality, etc.).
- ☐ I am open to conversations about mental health and well-being.
- ☐ I approach life at a relaxed pace, even when others seem rushed.
- ☐ I make time for creative or meditative activities.
- ☐ I am able to let go of things that are out of my control.
- ☐ I feel energised when I'm doing what I love, regardless of the outcome.

Score: _______

Scoring and interpretation

- Count the number of statements you checked in each part. Each box counts as one point. Your score reveals your current relationship with time.
- A higher score in Part 1 suggests a more time-anxious mindset, influenced by the external clock and a sense of restriction.

→

- A higher score in Part 2 suggests you have a more time-aligned mindset influenced by your own internal clock and a sense of abundance.
- Seeing where you resist or align helps you recognise how time itself can become part of your *rasāyana* journey so you can support vitality rather than drain it.

Āyurvedic concept 8: Western mechanisms and the *Āyurvedic* mirror

This chapter would not be complete without bridging the *Āyurvedic* understanding of health and ageing with modern science. What does contemporary research tell us about how we age? Modern theories echo *Āyurveda's* understanding of the body's complexity and interconnectedness, and its insight into balance and root causes. Here is a brief overview of the modern mechanics of ageing as I understand it.

DNA damage and repair decline

Your DNA carries the body's instructions, much like your *prakṛti* in *Āyurveda*. Over time, small errors and damage can build up from oxidative stress, toxins or replication errors during cell division. This leads to weakened repair, faster ageing and higher risk of disease. Though you're born with your genes, how well they function can change over time – like *vikṛti*.

The deadly disrupter – chronic inflammation

Inflammation is the body's natural and essential response to injury and to fight an infection, but when it becomes chronic, it fuels ageing at a cellular level. 'Inflammaging' is a type of persistent low-grade inflammation that accelerates tissue degeneration, leading to fatigue, brain fog, joint pain and basically 'feeling crap' and consequently can lead to chronic diseases, neurodegeneration, cardiovascular disease and metabolic disorders (e.g. diabetes). Often silent, chronic inflammation is one of the biggest culprits in premature ageing and is primarily caused by lifestyle choices. Chronic inflammation mirrors *Āyurveda's* mechanics of *pittā* aggravation (excess heat) and *āma* accumulation (toxins) that irritate and damage tissues over time.

Epigenetic changes

Your genotype is your fixed genetic code. Your phenotype reflects how that code is expressed and is not fixed. Environmental factors like food, stress, sleep and trauma influence gene expression, effectively acting like a dimmer switch that turns gene activity up or down without changing the DNA sequence itself. These changes affect the gene function and influence your health or disease. This is mirrored as a timeless truth in *Āyurveda*, which understands that diet and lifestyle constantly shapes your biological end game.

Oxidative stress

Every cell in your body uses oxygen. In that process, unstable molecules called free radicals are created. If they're not neutralised, they damage cells, much like rust on metal. This contributes to wrinkles, disease and faster ageing. Oxidative stress reflects the depletion of *ojas* and fading of *tejas*, weakening the body's ability to repair and protect itself.

Stem cell decline

Stem cells repair and regenerate tissues, keeping the body resilient. As you age, these cells become less active and, in most tissues, lose their ability to function properly even though their numbers may not decline. This slows healing, weakens tissue repair and raises the risk of degeneration. The body's in-built renewal system wears down over time. Stem cell decline mirrors the *Āyurvedic* picture of ***dhātu*** *and* ***ojas kṣaya*** the gradual depletion of tissues and reduced regeneration.

Telomere shortening

Telomeres are protective caps on the ends of your DNA (like indoor slippers). Each time a cell divides, telomeres shorten. When they get too short, the cell stops working or dies. Shorter telomeres are linked to faster ageing and chronic illness. This resembles premature ageing due to chronic *vāta* aggravation and long-term stress.

Mitochondrial dysfunction

Mitochondria are your cells' energy factories. Ageing damages them, reducing your ability to produce energy. This causes fatigue, brain fog and poor organ function. Mitochondrial decline is central to many age-related diseases. We can see *Āyurvedic* parallels with weak *agni* at the tissue (*dhātvagni*) level, resulting in poor cellular energy and vitality.

Metabolic dysregulation

Your body uses signals to decide when to burn or store energy. When these pathways go off-track, often due to overeating or irregular habits, it leads to weight gain, insulin resistance and accelerated ageing. We can correlate this to an impaired *agni* (metabolic fire) producing faulty ***rasa dhātu*** (plasma).

Protein damage

Proteins build and repair the body. As you age, some of them fold the wrong way or stick together in harmful clumps. These faulty proteins can disrupt how cells work and are linked to diseases like Alzheimer's, Parkinson's and other signs of degeneration.

Glycation and AGE (advanced glycation end-products)

When excess sugar binds to proteins, it creates sticky, damaging compounds that harden tissues and speed up ageing. This process of glycation is linked to wrinkles, diabetes and organ damage. It is seen in *Āyurveda* as the accumulation of *āma* in various body tissues such as *rakta* (blood) and *māṃsa* (muscle).

Senescent cells

These are damaged cells that no longer divide but refuse to die. They hang around, releasing harmful chemicals that affect neighbouring cells and promote inflammation and ageing. They're sometimes called 'zombie cells'. In *Āyurveda* this is similar to accumulation of *āma* (toxins) in the tissues.

Metabolic syndrome and chronic disease

A cluster of conditions, such as high blood pressure, insulin resistance and belly fat, speed up biological ageing and increase the risk of chronic disease. They're often the result of long-term lifestyle imbalance.

The concepts in this chapter show that natural ageing in Āyurveda is shaped by many interwoven forces. As we grow older, *vāta*, *agni*, *ojas*, *prāṇa*, *āma*, *dhātus*, *srotas*, *manas* and even our sense of connection are all in motion. They influence each other like the threads of a cloth. *Rasāyana* works by tending to all of them simultaneously so we can age with grace.

4

Ageing as a path for self-actualisation

'Realisation is not acquisition of anything new, nor is it a new faculty. It is only the removal of all camouflage.'

Ramana Maharshi

Why are you really here?

Let's pause for a moment. A strange way to start the chapter, I know! But I want you to ponder this as a priority: *Why are you here?*

I don't mean to read this book, but *here* – alive, breathing, on this planet, at this exact moment in time and space. What are your deepest desires? What do you long for? And what does a *good* life look like to you? What brings you a sense of fulfilment, success, happiness, healthfulness? Take as long as you need here – allow yourself the space to observe what is stirring within you. We all carry silent longings: some we fulfil, some we express, some we bury and some we outright deny ourselves.

These longings aren't random. That's your soul communicating through clues, sometimes subtle, sometimes screaming, about what truly matters to us. If we pay attention, they can show us what we're really here for.

In *Āyurveda*, a life well-lived begins with understanding the soul's journey. And that starts with one word: *purpose*. When purpose infuses our days, *rasāyana* becomes more than a process for well-being: it becomes a *way of* being. This chapter is focused on understanding how the soul grows as we mature.

We will examine:

- The four aims of life, or ***purushārthas***: ***dharma***, *ārtha,* ***kāma*** and ***mokṣa***
- How to make a sacred vow to your self – a ***saṅkalpa***
- How to shift from a victim to a visionary health mindset
- The four acts, or ***āśramas***, of life
- The five dimensions of your human being – the five *kośas*
- The concept of ageing as a sacred journey.

Studies show that living with a strong sense of purpose enhances both longevity and quality of life. It has been linked to lower rates of heart disease, reduced inflammation, better sleep and even sharper cognitive function as we age – a truth long understood by ancient *ācāryas*.

But beyond the data and headlines, our purpose, our *raison d'être*, is what puts the zest into our life, into our every day. Without it, life can feel directionless, like we're drifting rather than steering, disconnected from ourselves and the world around us.

The questions above are an invitation for you to turn inwards, to contemplate and slowly reconnect with who you truly are, and I don't mean the roles you play, the titles you hold, the identities that you've inherited – I mean who you are *beyond* all of that. Why have you arrived in this human earth suit? What if your health and well-being are intimately connected to how closely you live in alignment with that truth? Let's allow some time for that to marinate and then we'll come back to this again in pillar 7. Meanwhile, this leads us naturally to widen the lens and look at *Āyurveda's* framework for living well: the four aims of life.

The four aims of life: a blueprint for wholeness

धर्मार्थकाममोक्षाणामारोग्यं मूलमुत्तमम्।

dharmārtha-kāma-mokṣāṇām ārogyaṁ mūlam uttamam ||

'Health is the supreme foundation of *dharma*, *ārtha*, *kāma* and mokṣa.'

Caraka Saṃhitā, Sūtrasthāna 1.15

Āyurveda doesn't separate health from life. It sees health *as life* itself! Health is not the destination: it is the foundation. *Ācārya* Caraka frames health as the pathway to spiritual liberation and *rasāyana* is the *means* to sustain that journey.

Only when we have harmony in body and mind can we walk the deeper path of life – one of purpose, joy, prosperity and, ultimately, liberation.

In Vedic philosophy, a human life is said to have four essential aims, known as the *purushārthas* – a combination of two Sanskrit words: ***purusha***, meaning 'consciousness', 'spirit' or 'subtle human essence' and *ārtha,* meaning 'purpose', 'goal' or 'objective'. These are not check boxes, religious ideals or milestones to achieve, but rather living principles that help us navigate life with balance, meaning and direction.

When one of these areas is ignored or unfulfilled or another overindulged, imbalances arise and our health can suffer, in a similar way to how *doṣas* (three vital bio-energies, *see* pp. 39–43) get imbalanced in the body. If relationships or finances become strained, vitality can fade. But when the *purushārthas* are in harmony, our whole being buzzes with

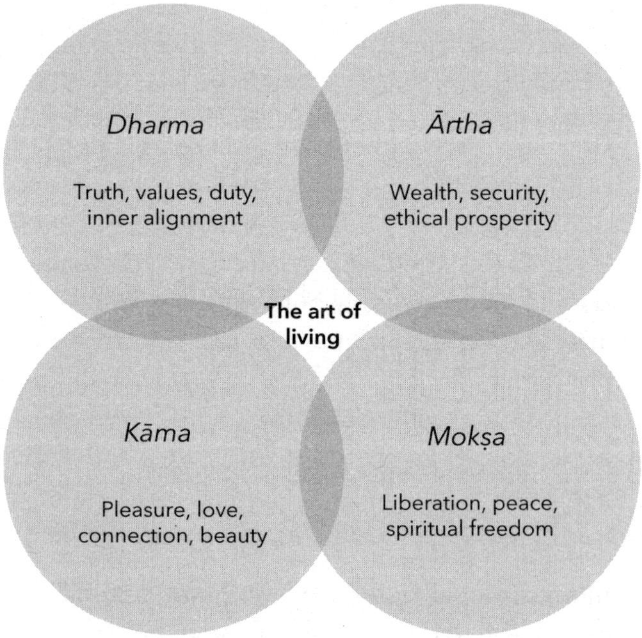

Figure 4.1 The Four Aims of Life (*purushārthas*)

vitality. Regardless of your religious background or belief system, there is one universal truth – we are all human, and we are all seeking meaning. And while we are in this body, we each deserve a life that is fulfilling and joyful. Before we build on your personal path and purpose, let's first explore each of the *purushārthas* and how they shape a life well-lived.

1. *Dharma* – your inner compass

Dharma is often oversimplified as religion, duty, purpose or 'doing the right thing' but in Vedic tradition, *dharma* is far more nuanced. At the highest level, *dharma* means alignment with the cosmic order – living in alignment with the flow of time, nature and truth.

When we speak of our personal path or ***svadharma***, it's not about choosing a job you like or following moral rules, it's about living in alignment with your unique purpose, your ethical values and your natural rhythm. It is living your 'truth'.

It's waking up each day with clarity, integrity and taking responsible steps in every part of life. A life guided by *dharma* brings emotional steadiness, softens stress and enhances resilience, contributing to both lifespan and healthspan.

I didn't uncover my true *dharma* until I was 27, when I formally embarked on my *Āyurveda* journey, not as a profession, but as a calling to serve humanity. It felt deeply aligned from the outset, as though it was a realisation just waiting to be downloaded. It wasn't a decision driven by money, status or a need to escape a marketing career: it felt like a subtle inner knowing that I simply had to follow. To this day, I never tire of it. I continue to learn, serve and grow through it. It energises rather than depletes me and I'm never just waiting for the weekend. I love it with the kind of certainty that only purpose can bring.

We all have a unique path and the realising of it brings a sense of deep fulfilment. It may not be blindingly obvious: it often appears as subtle signs through stillness, other times through challenge or curiosity. We will look at ways to identify your *dharma* in pillar 7.

2. *Ārtha* – the foundation of stability

We cannot meditate if we're hungry or stressed about paying the bills. ***Ārtha***, the pursuit of wealth and resources, is a sacred aim when it sustains life, not at the cost of it. As Maslow highlights in his Hierachy of Needs, self-actualisation can only be attained when our basic needs are not in a struggle.

True *ārtha* supports the wellness of self, family and your community. Material stability allows us to access quality healthcare, nourishing food and safe living conditions. But when material pursuits turn into greed or endless acquisition, we instead manifest burnout, disease and disconnection.

3. *Kāma* – the art of joyful living

Kāma is often reduced to the desire for and the act of sexual pleasure, which is commonly viewed as taboo, sinful or shameful. But *kāma* is neither limited to sexual pleasure nor sinful – it's sacred. It's a gift of being born in a human body, with sensory organs designed to experience beauty, connection, joy and love – we can learn to take better care of our senses through pillar 6. When we honour this mindfully, *kāma* is not indulgence, it's a celebration of life itself and it plays a vital role in our well-being. In fact, modern research shows that people who experience love, intimacy and belonging tend to live longer and healthier lives.

What's the principle of pleasure? Not to *deny* it, but to enjoy it *wisely in the moment*, neither to develop a dependency nor depression in the not having of it. It fuels rather than depletes health and harmony. Uncontrolled indulgences for short-term gratification, however, can be the precursor to many kinds of addictions that lead to diseases.

4. *Mokṣa* – the ultimate liberation

Mokṣa is ultimate freedom, not just from suffering, but from illusions (*māyā*) that keep us entangled in false identities and worldly attachments (*viṣaya*). It is a realisation that we are not limited to the body, role or story but we're inseparable from consciousness or the oneness. This is the unveiling of the quest for self-actualisation and the question: 'Who am I?' This is the root of ***Advaita Vedānta***, the non-dualism tradition of the Upanishads and reinforced by the teachings of the late sage, Ramana Maharshi. It's a deep exhale, a coming home to your true self. It's found through meditation, silence, self-inquiry and the simple act of letting go, which we explore in pillar 7.

In health, *mokṣa* means we don't just manage physical symptoms, we explore the deeper roots and seek healing on the soul level.

In pursuit of *mokṣa*, we can subsequently reduce stress, improve mental clarity and foster a sense of purpose, all of which help us age well. Pro-ageing is not about defying age: it's about deepening through it.

The more grounded and nourished your body and mind, the more capacity you have for clarity, intuition and spiritual expansion. So, to honour the body is to honour the path of evolution. Remember, health is your birthright and the stepping stone for spiritual evolution. While the *purushārthas* offer us a roadmap to life, a *saṅkalpa* provides us with a compass that helps us walk our path with a soul-aligned intention.

A sacred vow to self

Let me share an exercise I do with most of my clients, because healing and pro-ageing begins with intentionality: *saṅkalpa*.

Unlike a goal, which comes from the agenda of our ego, a *saṅkalpa* arises from deep within. It is a sacred vow to your higher self – allowing us to age with *intention*. We make promises and vows to others all the time, often without a second thought; we even take big risks to enter binding contracts such as marriages and buying homes. But let me ask you this, and please take a moment here – when did you last (or ever) make a committed vow to yourself?

Unlike the short-term intentions at the start of a yoga class, a *saṅkalpa* helps align your daily choices, boundaries, habits and goals with your deeper purpose (*dharma*), guiding your decisions so you're not pulled in different directions, but moving forwards with clarity. Your *saṅkalpa* may be kept for months, even years, until your direction changes. A *saṅkalpa* might sound like:

- *I am vibrant. I am at peace. I am aligned*
- *I am curious, connected and evolving every day*
- *I nourish my body, protect my energy and walk in rhythm with nature*
- *I vow to care for my mind with kindness, prioritising rest, nourishment and joy*
- *I am courageous, compassionate and overflowing with vitality.*

A *saṅkalpa* is simple, powerful and in the present tense.

Create your *saṅkalpa* - a sacred intention

1. Sit quietly for a few minutes, breathing deeply to connect with yourself.
2. Ask: *How do I need to show up for myself? What brings me into deep alignment?*
3. Let your intention arise from within, not from fear or outside expectations.
4. Form a short, clear statement in the present tense that aligns deeply.
5. Speak it aloud, visualise it and feel it in your body as a truth.
6. Repeat your *saṅkalpa* daily, letting it guide your thoughts, choices and actions.
7. Live in alignment with this intention. Let it shape how you spend your time and energy.

Repeat your *saṅkalpa* each morning; let it be your guiding star. You can think of your *saṅkalpa* as the mission statement of your life - a soulful real-time declaration that helps you live in alignment with or towards your *dharma*.

Shifting from victim to visionary health mindset

I pay close attention to the words my clients use to describe themselves and their health concerns: the tone behind their stories, the language they choose, their facial expressions, the silences and pauses, and their body language that speaks a thousand words. It reveals so much more than knowing the symptoms alone (we explore this more in pillar 5). It helps me understand the mindset that may have contributed to their current state and how best to guide their healing journey ahead, especially when deeper ***saṃskāras*** (subconscious impressions) are influencing their current health issues (*see* pillar 7). But for now, have you noticed how you speak about yourself and your health?

When I invite clients to reflect on how they've been speaking about their health, I usually notice that they're seeing themselves as helpless or stuck, followed quickly by a moment of realisation. They begin to recognise how their narrative isn't just describing their health; it's shaping it. The Revd. Dr Michael Beckwith's four stages of consciousness lends a modern map of spiritual evolution echoing themes found in Vedantic texts, reflecting mindset shifts we may experience repeatedly in different areas of life. These are:

1. *Life happens* to me – *I am a victim.*
2. *Life happens* by me – *I am an active participant. I take responsibility.*
3. *Life flows* through me – *I surrender to higher guidance.*
4. *Life happens* as me – *I* am *life. I live in oneness.*

Through my health coaching, I see how these states of consciousness profoundly shape how we relate to our health and to our outlook on ageing. In the West, most people live in the 'to me' phase, outsourcing health to systems and experts – we slip into 'self-gaslighting' mode, invalidate our intuition and deny our power to heal ourselves. *Āyurveda* encourages us to move beyond 'to me' into the 'by me' and 'through me' phases, and ultimately towards 'as me', like a co-creator of life aligned with our soul and nature.

True transformation happens as we gently unlearn the negative habits and beliefs we've unknowingly picked up. Once we drown out the noise, we can hear our intuitive voice, regain self-trust and reclaim our agency. The question is, how much do you want to reclaim sovereignty over your own health?

A life in four acts

Life doesn't come with a map, so we're all just fumbling through, but when it comes to our *wellness*, we don't need to. The Vedic sages gave us a framework of four distinct stages of life, called the *āśramas.* We're not meant to live in the same way at every age. Our health, rituals and priorities evolve, and *Āyurveda* guides us to adapt to the seasons of our life.

Modern wellness culture often defies this flow. We're taught to fear ageing, glorify youth and pathologise change. What if 'retirement' wasn't something we waited for, but something we practised in small ways throughout life? What if we regularly paused to reflect, reset and realign? Surely this would give us a chance to check in with ourselves to see what's nourishing us and what's not.

Let's take a closer look at each of these four stages which guide us towards a more conscious way of ageing.

Āśramas	**Key features**
Brahmacharya (0–25 years) The season of becoming	A time of learning, curiosity, building discipline and strong life skills. Personal identity begins to emerge. Daily habits around food, sleep and movement lay the foundations for resilience.
Gṛhastha (25–50 years) The season of creation	These householder years are vibrant and expansive, focusing on relationships, career, children and worldly contribution. *Āyurveda* recognises the pressures of this phase, so guides us to pro-age by protecting our energy with daily rituals, rest and nourishment to avoid burnout. Beginning *rasāyana* practices at this time is a huge bonus.
Vānaprastha (50–75 years) The season of wisdom	A gentle turning inwards begins. This is a time to gently transition from doing to being. Shifting from the hustle mode to simplicity and wisdom. This is the time for focused *rasāyana* practices, deeper self-inquiry and being guided by nature.
Sannyāsa (75-plus years) The season of stillness	The final stage calls for material detachment, deep contemplation and inner peace. Health is measured by presence, not productivity. The body thrives with softness, stillness, spiritual maturity. *Rasāyana* practices and herbs are integral.

Table 4.1 The four *āśramas*

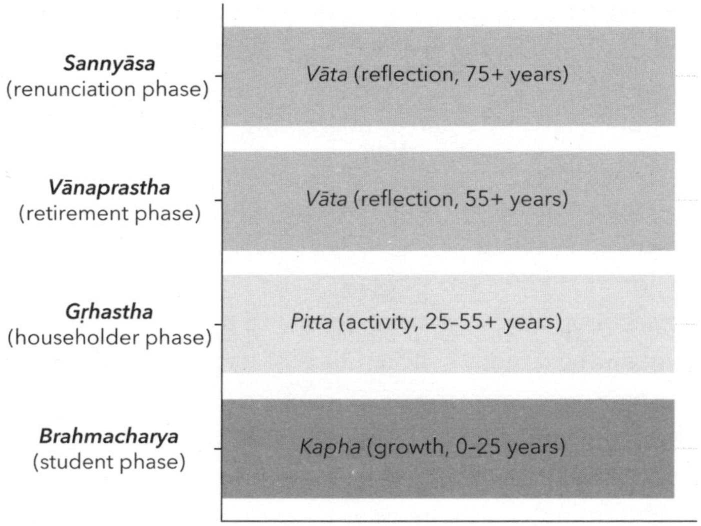

Figure 4.2 The four *āśramas* mapped to *doṣas* and age groups

Let's ask a few reflective questions here:

- What do you expect to happen when you 'retire'?
- How would you invest your time, money and energy?
- What activities or people would you prioritise?
- What passions would you nurture?
- What is the legacy that you want to leave behind?
- What's stopping you from starting some or all these things now?

Five dimensions of your human being

Remember those Russian nesting dolls, each one opening to reveal another inside? You're built the same way. Beneath your physical form lie four more subtle layers of being, each one more refined than the last. And at your core? The soul, or *ātman*.

You are a whole being - not just a body, but energy, emotion, intuition and spirit. True pro-ageing means creating harmony at all of these layers so they can work together in harmony. These ***pañca kośas*** (five sheaths) influence how you live, how you heal, how you age.

In many Eastern cultures, especially in India, ageing isn't feared, it's revered. Elders are seen as wisdom keepers, not relics. Their presence is greatly honoured and their stories devoured. This layered view of human existence helps us reframe ageing as a privilege instead of a decline.

When your body's tired, your mind's restless or your spirit's disconnected, your layers are misaligned and true well-being feels out of reach, no matter how many supplements or treatments you try. But when you tend to every layer, from the most visible to the most subtle, something shifts. You tap into an embodied power and vitality can flourish – the seven pillars in part 2 will help you tap into and nourish all the layers of your being, starting from the gross level to the subtle as we progress. So, what are the five *kośas* and how do they relate to well-being?

The *pañca kośa*

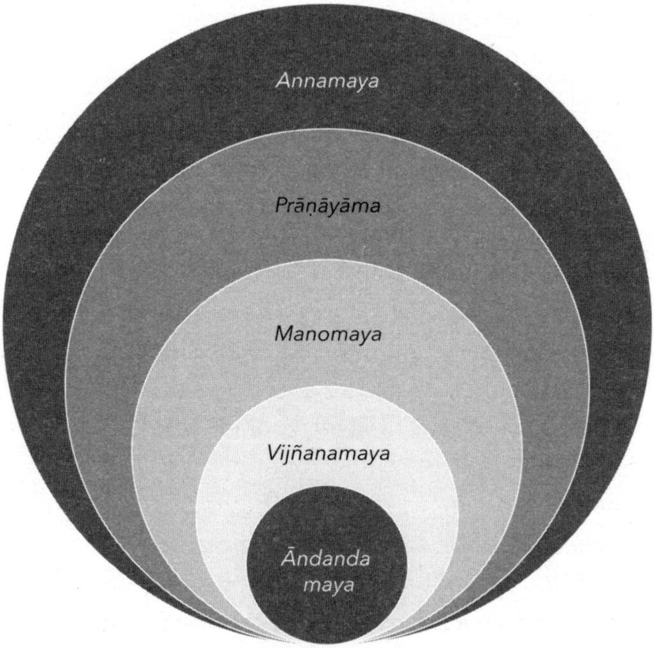

Figure 4.3 The five *kośas*

1. *Annamaya kośa* (physical body)

The outermost layer is the visible, physical body. Shaped by what you eat, how you move and the rhythms you live by, it reflects your everyday choices. Rooted in ***pṛthvī*** (earth energy), this *kośa* feels grounded through simplicity and self-care. Nourish it with *sattvic* food, good sleep and steady movement to support strength, immunity and lasting vitality.

2. *Prāṇamaya kośa* (energy body)

This is your subtle body of breath and life force, *prāṇa*, which animates and energises the physical form. Flowing through the *nādīs* (subtle energy channels) and ***marma*** points, it connects breath, movement and vitality. Associated with water (***jala***), it reflects fluidity and flow. Practices like *prāṇāyāma* (breathwork and energy regulation), gentle yoga and energy healing can help manage stress, support oxygenation and restore balance.

3. *Manomaya kośa* (mental body)

The emotional and mental layer is home to our memories, emotions and sensory perception. Governed by fire (*agni*), it shapes how we perceive and respond to life. We can regulate emotions through meditation and mindfulness, while inner child healing, 'shadow work' (*see* p. 238) and stress management support cognitive clarity, stabilise emotions and promote long-term mental well-being.

4. *Vijñānamaya kośa* (intelligence body)

This is the sheath of intellect, compassion, discernment and higher wisdom. When balanced, it helps us stay calm, clear and focused beyond the drama of the ego. Associated with air (***vayu***), this *kośa* thrives through reflection, learning and nourishing relationships. Practices like visualisation and somatic work (a movement- and sensations-based practice to regulate the nervous system and release stored stress) enhance neuroplasticity and purpose.

5. *Ānandamaya kośa* (bliss body)

Ānanda means 'bliss' – our truest natural state of pure consciousness. This sheath reflects harmony, bliss and connection to our deeper soul (*ātman*). This all-pervasive *kośa* is associated with space (*ākāśa*). Practices like meditation, devotional chanting, connection with nature, and acts of kindness awaken peace and a deeper sense of fulfilment.

By embracing all layers of our being and integrating practices that nurture vitality and slow degeneration, this framework provides a holistic path to age consciously.

A rite of passage – ageing as a sacred journey

Ageing (***jarā***) is a slow and natural process of physical and mental changes and over time we may see an increase in our vulnerability to diseases and, eventually, death. There, I've said it, that dreaded word that always feels so taboo. But surely, we should be able to talk about and embrace the inevitable? After all, *memento mori* – 'remember that you must die' – is not a morbid thought, but a gentle truth found across many traditions, from Latin Stoic philosophy to the Vedic concept of ***anitya*** (impermanence). If we remembered how fleeting life is more often, then maybe we would live more fully every day.

In Vedic philosophy, ageing is seen as a rite of passage, an opportunity to embody wisdom, rather than being doomed from womb to tomb. If we can maintain proper balance, the later stages of life can be just as meaningful, purposeful and joyful as our youth. Health becomes the long game; the foundation that supports a fulfilling life and the pursuit of the four aims of life or *purushārthas*. It's not about chasing youth, but choosing *pro-ageing*, supporting life with rhythm, care and intention.

This understanding isn't exclusive to *Āyurveda*. In Yoruba wisdom, there's a saying (paraphrased here): 'A person who does not remember where they came from will not reach where they are going.' Ageing is not just physical, it's ancestral, spiritual and relational. Similarly, the Q'ero shamans of the Andes view death not as an end but as a sacred portal. Their *Amauta* teachings remind us that to live well is to honour cycles of birth, decay, renewal and to walk in *ayni* – sacred reciprocity with time, nature and spirit.

Dutch theosophist JJ van der Leeuw said, 'The mystery of life is not a problem to be solved, but a reality to be experienced.' Ageing brings home this truth. It asks us to participate more deeply and fully show up, today and every day.

Death takes no prisoners and contemplating death alone rarely sparks a change in health. We delay, we plan, we wait for the 'right time'. As American Buddhist teacher and author Jack Kornfield, and commonly misattributed to the Buddha once said: 'The trouble is, you think you have time.' Knowing this, the real question is not *when* we will die, but *how* we will live. The way to embrace the richness of now and at the same time future-proof your life and close the 'vitality gap' is simple: start today. You don't need to do everything at once: choose one thing that nurtures vitality and start there – move your body, strengthen your digestion, calm your mind, connect with someone you love.

A bedtime story: 'The Princess and the Old Man'

Long ago, a king's daughter refused every suitor, so the king created a test. Blindfolded, she would choose her husband by touch. As fate would have it, her hand landed on an elderly holy man delivering herbs in the courtyard. Though he protested, the king insisted on honouring the choice.

Distressed, the old man turned to his teacher, who prescribed a strict 90-day *kāya-kalpa* regimen with restorative herbs, nourishing foods, oil massages and yogic practices. With discipline, he followed it all. Slowly, his hair darkened, his skin softened, his vitality returned.

By the end of the 90 days, he was transformed – radiant, strong and youthful. When he returned to the palace, the princess was stunned and overjoyed. Their marriage blossomed, and their story became a legend.

The story invites us to see that true youthfulness comes from within as well as through the rejuvenating power of *rasāyana*.

5

Gut healthy first

'One cannot think well, love well, sleep well, if one has not dined well.'

***A Room of One's Own*, Virginia Woolf**

In this chapter, we begin where all transformation starts: the gut. We lay the foundation for *rasāyana* by preparing the body and mind through *laṅghana* (lightening or cleansing). Before we flood the body with nourishment, the very essence of *rasāyana*, we must first make space for it. Think of it as a 'factory reset' allowing your phone to function more smoothly. *Laṅghana* is not a trendy detox but a deeply rooted *Āyurvedic* process that clears the toxins (*āma*) that do not serve, so that we can fully absorb what does.

In this chapter, we explore practical ways to prepare you for *rasāyana* by:

- Mindful eating rituals and *laṅghana* practices to clear toxins and promote gut health
- ***Dīpana*** and ***pācana*** (kindling and cleansing digestion)
- Fasting methods to reset your gut
- Hydration wisdom to keep digestion balanced.

But let's first understand why this process is essential.

Why we 'lighten' before *rasāyana*

When our *agni* (digestive fire) is sluggish, *āma* (undigested metabolic residue) begins to accumulate, further dulling *agni* and disrupting the body's ability to process not only food, but also thoughts, emotions and experiences. Over time, this leads to stagnation - physically, mentally and energetically.

To break this cycle, *Āyurveda* turns to *laṅghana,* the classical practice of 'lightening' the body and mind. By clearing *āma* and rekindling *agni*, *laṅghana* restores the body's natural clarity, vitality and readiness to rejuvenate. You cannot nourish a system that's already overloaded – just as you wouldn't pour fresh water into a contaminated vessel to drink from.

At the physical level, *agni* is the body's powerhouse of transformation: breaking down food, absorbing nutrients, generating energy and eliminating waste. When *agni* is steady, you feel clear, light, energised and resilient. When it's weak or imbalanced, you may feel heavy, bloated, foggy or fatigued, even if you're eating a wholesome diet.

Without a well-functioning *agni*, *rasāyana* practices, no matter how nourishing, cannot be properly digested, absorbed or integrated. Instead, they may give rise to further *āma*. That's why this chapter begins with one essential task: restoring and strengthening your *agni*, especially when it's *manda* (dull), *viṣama* (irregular) or *tīkṣṇa* (too sharp). Rebalancing *agni* not only enhances rejuvenation through the seven pillars but to essentially help reduce *āma* and cool chronic inflammation – one of the key drivers of accelerated ageing and age-related conditions.

In practice, *laṅghana* may involve fasting, lighter meals, resting the gut, staying hydrated or using gentle herbs. By easing the digestive load and creating inner space, *laṅghana* sets the stage for the body to receive nourishment on a deeper level.

Before we dive into these practices, it helps to pause and see where your digestion stands right now. The '*agni* health self-check' below is a simple tool to help you identify what your body may be signalling, so let's get straight to belly business.

Agni health self-check

To help you identify signs of balanced or imbalanced *agni* in your daily life, reflect on each question and answer honestly (tick all that apply to you).

Signs of balanced agni

- ☐ I feel genuine hunger before meals; I'm not just eating out of habit or boredom.

→

- ☐ I feel satisfied yet light after eating, not heavy, bloated or sluggish.
- ☐ My bowel movements are regular, well formed and easy to pass.
- ☐ I rarely experience gas, bloating, indigestion or burping.
- ☐ My energy levels are steady and consistent, without crashing or feeling wired after meals.
- ☐ I eat at consistent times and complete digestion within four to six hours.
- ☐ I am able to adjust to and tolerate seasonal changes.
- ☐ I have little to no odour from stools or breath.
- ☐ My tongue feels clean and free from a thick coating.
- ☐ After eating, I feel clear-headed, emotionally balanced and at ease.

Signs of imbalanced *agni*

- ☐ I tend to feel heavy, bloated or sluggish after meals.
- ☐ I have a sensitive digestion / indigestion / intolerance to certain foods.
- ☐ My elimination varies and I could have constipation, loose stools or difficulty passing stools.
- ☐ I frequently experience gas, bloating or discomfort.
- ☐ My energy spikes and crashes after eating, or I can feel drowsy or anxious.
- ☐ I need stimulants (coffee, tea, sugar) to get going in the morning.
- ☐ I wake up feeling unrested, even after a good sleep or lethargic in the day.
- ☐ I have a coating on my tongue, most mornings.
- ☐ I have an erratic appetite, insatiable hunger or sometimes no hunger at all.
- ☐ I feel foggy-headed, moody or uneasy after eating.

What is your *agni* telling you?

If you've ticked more signs of imbalance, don't worry. This chapter offers guidance, insight and gentle practices to help reduce *āma*, reset your system and bring your *agni* back into balance.

If your *agni* already feels strong and balanced, stay with me! There's still much to discover. Even if your *agni* is balanced, this chapter will help you deepen your intuition and refine your everyday habits. So, whether you're clearing the way or fine-tuning your fire, this chapter is essential to set the stage for lasting renewal.

In all the noise, we've forgotten the one golden rule of *Āyurveda*: what matters most is not *what* you eat, but *how* you digest, and this is why we pay so much attention to maintaining a balanced *agni*. Poor digestion of even the healthiest food can lead to *āma* that subsequently clogs the body's channels. On the other hand, well-digested simple meals, cooked with care and eaten mindfully, become medicine.

एवं विशुद्धकोष्ठस्य कायाग्निरभिवर्धते।
व्याधयश्चोपशाम्यन्ति प्रकृतिश्चानुवर्तते॥
इन्द्रियाणि मनोबुद्धिर्वर्णश्चास्य प्रसीदति।
बलं पुष्टिरपत्यं च वृषता चास्य जायते॥
जरां कृच्छ्रेण लभते चिरं जीवत्यनामयः।
तस्मात् संशोधनं काले युक्तियुक्तं पिबेन्नरः॥

evaṃ viśuddhakoṣṭhasya kāyāgnir abhivardhate |
vyādhayaś copaśāmyanti prakṛtiś cānuvartate ||
indriyāṇi mano buddhir varṇaś cāsya prasīdati |
balaṃ puṣṭir apatyam ca vṛṣatā cāsya jāyate ||
jarāṃ kṛcchreṇa labhate ciraṃ jīvati anāmayaḥ |
tasmāt saṃśodhanaṃ kāle yuktiyuktaṃ pibet naraḥ ||

'When the digestive system is purified properly, digestive fire strengthens, diseases subside, and the natural balance is restored. Clarity of mind, senses and intellect improves along with vitality and strength. Ageing slows, and one lives long and free from disease. Therefore, purification should be undertaken at the proper time and in the right way.'

Caraka Saṃhitā, Sūtrasthāna 16. 17–19

Laṅghana beyond the gut

Your liver, kidneys, lungs, colon, skin and lymphatic system are working hard every day to detoxify and protect you, so what they crave is support, not sabotage. *Laṅghana* practices lighten the load, gently cleansing and allowing your body's natural detox systems to do what they're designed to do.

Although we predominately speak about *laṅghana* in relation to the gut and *agni*, its scope is wider. *Laṅghana* is also about calming the mind and clearing the senses and letting go of what's emotionally or energetically weighing us down. We'll explore these dimensions more deeply in pillars 5, 6 and 7.

Daily *laṅghana* lifestyle tips

Here are gentle, everyday ways to lighten the system, support gut health and help prevent the build-up of *āma*. Don't feel pressured to do everything at once. Pick one or two practices to start today - whichever feel most natural or exciting to you. Over time, as your awareness deepens, you can layer in more until these habits truly feel like second nature:

- **Wake up and sleep in sync with the sun** - this helps maintain your body's natural bio-rhythms.
- **Start your day with a glass of plain warm water** - ginger, lemon, or a little **ghee** are optional additions, used as needed rather than as a daily habit (avoid lemon if prone to heartburn or acidity).
- **Make lunch your main meal of the day** - this is when your *agni* is naturally strongest.
- **Avoid snacking between meals** - give your digestion time to rest and reset.
- **Integrate digestive spices into your food and drinks** - such as cumin, coriander, fennel, ginger, carom, black pepper.
- **Ensure you move gently every day** - walking or yoga encourages healthy lymph flow.
- **Practise deep conscious breathing** - stillness brings calm to the mind and emotions.
- **Manage your portion sizes** - fill half the stomach with food, a quarter with water and leave a quarter empty so digestion happens most efficiently.
- **Eat consciously** - focus on your food. Avoid distractions such as screens, multitasking or eating on the go.
- **Opt for warm, fresh meals** - avoid cold, stale or ultra-processed food.
- **Slow down, chew well** - because digestion begins in both the mouth and the mind.
- **Skip the icy drinks** - especially before, during or after meals.
- **Eat only when you genuinely feel hunger** - keep on top of your hunger cues: don't force it, don't ignore it.

→

- **Watch out for signs of imbalance** – such as bloating, gas, belching and acidity, which can indicate disturbed *agni*. Seek out professional help if you have persistent gastro-intestinal issues.

These simple acts, done with consistency, are the real magic behind feeling clear, light and energised that prepare your body to receive foods that nourish (pillar 2).

Stimulating the digestive fire

While we continue to integrate daily *laṅghana* lifestyle practices for our general gut health, our digestive fire, or *agni*, sometimes needs more focused attention. When *agni* feels sluggish, irregular or overwhelmed by *āma*, you might feel heavy, foggy or bloated, even with healthy habits in place. In *Āyurveda*, this is where *dīpana* and *pācana* play a role in restoring gut health.

- *Dīpana* means 'kindling *agni*'. It stimulates and awakens your digestive flame so it can digest well. It's helpful when appetite is low, digestion feels dull or food feels like it just sits in the stomach.
- *Pācana* means 'digesting *āma*' or burning away the existing toxins that clog your system.

Together, *dīpana* and *pācana* prepare your body for deeper cleansing or act as a gentle digestive reset during seasonal transitions or times of *āma* accumulation.

Simple *dīpana-pācana* practices

Here are four simple *dīpana-pācana* practices to help stoke your *agni* and clear *āma*. You can, but don't need to, do all of them, or just start with one or two that feel easy to add into your day. You can then stop when you feel your *agni* is back on track (use the '*agni* health self-check' on pp. 73–4).

1. Eat light, warming meals such as mung dal, soups, steamed vegetables or ***khichdi*** (kitchari - a lightly spiced *Āyurvedic* stew of rice and mung dal - *see* recipe, pp. 136–7).
2. Take a preparation of ½–1 tsp freshly grated ginger with a pinch of rock salt and a squeeze of lime, 15 minutes before meals.
3. Drink spiced herbal teas such as cumin-coriander-fennel (CCF, *see* recipe below) or ginger-black pepper-cinnamon. I also love simple carom seed (*ajwain)* tea.
4. Take a herbal formula - *trikatu cūrṇa* (in moderation) before meals if digestion is heavy or sluggish (consult your practitioner if symptoms persist).

These are subtle but powerful ways to restore metabolic efficiency and prime your system to be receptive to *rasāyana* foods and herbs.

CCF gut tea (cumin, coriander, fennel)

A gentle, daily digestive tea to kindle *agni* and flush *āma.* It supports gentle detoxification, reduces bloating and boosts digestion.

Makes about 1 litre

Ingredients:

- 1.25 litres water
- 1 tsp cumin seeds
- 1 tsp coriander seeds
- 1 tsp fennel seeds

Method:

1. Bring the water to the boil in a pan.
2. Add all three seeds - whole (or you can gently crush them first using a mortar and pestle to release more flavour and potency). I keep a jar of mixed seeds ready to go!
3. Reduce the heat and let the tea simmer, covered loosely, for four minutes for a mild brew, and for up to eight minutes for a strong brew.
4. Strain using a fine-mesh sieve.
5. Sip the tea warm, first thing in the morning, or between meals during the day (not with meals). You can store it in a flask to keep it warm throughout the day.

A periodic deep reset (*pañcakarma*)

While the *laṅghana* lifestyle and *dīpana-pācana* practices help maintain daily balance, sometimes the body gives us signals that a more thorough reset is needed, especially when *āma* has been accumulating over time, *doṣas* have become deeply imbalanced and you are subsequently dealing with chronic lifestyle conditions such as stubborn weight gain, chronic fatigue, skin conditions, recurring gut issues, hormonal imbalances, bone and joint stiffness, or anxiety. *Āyurveda* offers a more systemic therapeutic reset called *pañcakarma*, the 'five actions' of purification. These treatments are traditionally used to clear deeply embedded toxins, restore *agni* and reset the body's *doṣas* at a foundational level, after which the body is fully receptive and ready for *rasāyana*, herbs, nourishing foods, therapies and lifestyle to take effect.

Pañcakarma is *not* a home cleanse, but a periodic, purposeful and personalised intervention, often used as a precursor to the classical *kuti praveśikā rasāyana* protocols (*see* chapter 2). The five core therapies include:

1. ***Vamana*** - therapeutic vomiting to clear excess *kapha* (mucous and heaviness)
2. ***Virechana*** - purgation to clear excess *pitta* (heat and inflammation)
3. ***Basti*** - medicated enemas to calm and balance *vāta* and nourish the tissues
4. ***Nasya*** - nasal therapies to clear and support the head, sinuses and mind
5. ***Raktamokṣana*** - therapeutic blood cleansing for targeted conditions

Pañcakarma is a deep purification intervention that requires thorough preparation, supervision and post-procedure aftercare from a highly qualified and experienced *Āyurvedic* practitioner. Never attempt these procedures unsupervised at home. Consult your doctor if you have pre-existing health conditions.

→

If you feel in need of a deeper seasonal or supervised *pañcakarma*, it is best to contact an *Āyurvedic* practitioner - *see* the Resources section on pp. 271-2 for more details.

> **'A cleansed body without *rasāyana* is vulnerable. A rejuvenated body without cleansing is ineffective. Both must go hand in hand.'**
>
> **Geeta Vara**

Fasting for longevity

Fasting is a timeless practice, deeply ingrained in cultural and religious traditions across the globe. In India, practices like fasting on ***Ekādaśī*** (the 11th day of the lunar cycle) and *Navarātri* (a seasonal nine-day fast that falls in spring and autumn), and other spiritually significant days such as *Śivarātri* (night of devotion to Lord Shiva) and *Janmāṣṭamī* (celebration of the birth of Lord Krishna) have been followed for centuries. These fasting traditions make use of the seasonal transitions that naturally support cleansing and rebalancing of the body - interestingly the focus of fasting was to gain spiritual clarity by lightening (*laṅghana*) the diet or limiting the diet to specific foods, not necessarily total abstinence of food for long periods.

Similarly, in many cultures, fasting is woven into spiritual practice. The Islamic tradition of Ramadan, the Christian tradition of Lent and the Jewish practice of Yom Kippur all integrate fasting as a discipline for spiritual development. While most people will associate fasting with the religious aspect of their culture, what if I told you that beyond its spiritual and cultural significance, *Āyurvedic* fasting (as a *laṅghana* practice) holds the key to slowing down ageing?

Āyurveda has always advocated safe and appropriate fasting, known as *upavāsa*, as a tool to cleanse the body and mind for enhancing vitality, improving healthspan and promoting longevity. With growing public interest in longevity and the rising scientific research on fasting, *Āyurveda* offers wise, practical ways to use fasting in daily life to support better health and well-being. Fasting is not always appropriate for everyone; please *see* the box on p. 88 for contraindications.

Fasting is a cornerstone of preparation for *rasāyana* (rejuvenation therapy) and an integral component of *kuti praveśikā* (rejuvenation therapy during isolation in a hut), but how can we integrate a model that is equally safe and beneficial? Fasting is not a 'detox' or weight-loss hack: it's a natural rhythm of life, where periods of nourishment are balanced with rest for the digestive system. In *Āyurveda*, fasting is not a daily lifestyle strategy but a therapeutic tool used when digestion is overloaded (*āma*). Its purpose is to give our digestive and metabolic capacity (*agni*) a chance to recover. The fasting window is not set by the clock but by honouring true hunger.

Let's pause to explore the incredible mechanisms that fasting unleashes in the body – after all, I have to give you reasons to buy into the concept of fasting for *Āyurvedic* pro-ageing.

Autophagy: the body's clean-up crew

Modern science now reveals a biological miracle – that when our system is empty, the body shifts from processing food to repair mode. One process activated is autophagy – the body's cellular housekeeping, a Marie Kondo style tidy-up inside the cells, where damaged material is cleared and recycled.

When we are constantly eating, this repair function becomes less efficient. Periods without food allow the body to redirect energy towards maintenance and restoration.

Āyurveda describes a related process through ***āma pācana***, the digestion and clearing of accumulated metabolic residue when *agni* is no longer constantly processing food. Autophagy may be understood as one modern-day parallel of this process.

Fasting therefore gives the body a chance to shift into a repair state when necessary to support healthy ageing, so your biology can better keep up with your trips around the sun. However, when fasting is too intense or prolonged, it can deplete the body tissues, a condition Ayurveda calls *dhātu kṣhaya*.

Metabolic health

Āyurveda encourages eating only when there is genuine hunger and knowing the difference between feeling hungry, feeling full and feeling comfortably empty in between meals. In a modern scientific sense, we are developing a conscious connection with ghrelin (the hunger hormone) and leptin (the fullness hormone). Eating at regular intervals and not snacking between meals allows *agni* to fire up nice and strong in the run-up to a meal - i.e. the time to rest and digest, followed by a period of comfortable emptiness. *Āyurveda* also teaches us to complete our evening meal at least two to three hours before bed and to avoid or minimise heavy foods during the slow, heavy, grounded hours of *kapha* - between 6 and 10 a.m./p.m. (*see* p. 97 for diurnal clock). This means the body naturally goes through periods of fasting each day and our digestion naturally aligns with the energy of the sun.

This is mirrored in the modern ideas of 'time-restricted eating' and 'intermittent fasting', which have been shown to improve insulin sensitivity, reduce inflammation and lower the risk of chronic diseases like diabetes and cardiovascular conditions.

Disciplined eating patterns

For the past several years I've followed a simple routine of eating two main meals a day, finishing before or as close to 6 p.m. as possible and 'breaking fast' at around 10.30/11 a.m. Sure, there's flexibility for social commitments, but the benefits of a consistent daily fasting window are undeniable. The idea of fasting can feel daunting, especially if you've never tried it, but just like anything new, it becomes easier with guidance and practice. Yes, there's mild discomfort initially, a growling stomach here, a craving for a late-night snack there, but this can create a little *healthy* stress. With time, this discomfort transforms into clarity, energy and lightness; we simply require discipline and a little willpower to start provided it suits you. - *see* p. 88 for safety and contraindications.

Perhaps our mindset around fasting needs a shift. Instead of associating it with deprivation (which it is not), why not view it as a long-term investment in your body? Growing up, I witnessed my community participate in religious fasting rituals. While some followed these genuinely, others found many loopholes to justify indulgences for foods that 'are allowed'. The difference lies in intention. Fasting, when done with awareness, becomes effortless and joyful. Smaller portions, longer gaps between meals, mindful eating and occasional fasting seem to unlock remarkable vitality and longevity across the blue zone communities we looked at on p. 24.

When our body experiences periods of short-term fasting this induces mild (good) stress, activates the body's repair mechanisms and strengthens resilience, something known today as *hormesis*.

Eating within a shorter daily window gives your body longer breaks from food, so blood sugar and insulin levels can drop, and your body can use insulin more efficiently. This pattern may help to reduce insulin resistance and, over time, could lower type 2 diabetes risk, especially when most food is eaten earlier in the day. For those already struggling with blood sugar imbalances, fasting benefits can still be unleashed in a gentler way according to your constitution (*prakṛti*), current imbalance (*vikṛti*) and with close practitioner guidance, but *laṅghana* practices are a good and safe start.

Studies suggest that fasting increases brain-derived neurotrophic factor (BDNF), a protein essential for memory and learning and protection of brain cells. It also activates autophagy, the body's clean-up process. Emerging research in humans suggests that intermittent fasting can enhance markers of autophagy, and experimental work links this mechanism to cognitive resilience and the prevention of neurodegenerative pathology, a key area of study in brain-ageing research.

Why fasting matters more than ever

In a world where excess of anything is now the norm, many of our health challenges stem not from a lack of food but from overconsumption. Chronic inflammation, insulin resistance and the so-called 'diseases of affluence' can all stem from indulging in something over the limits of what our system can handle – known in *Āyurveda* as *prajñāparādha* (going against our own inner wisdom). Fasting opens our mind and body to a mini reset on a regular basis so we can find a way to restore balance and prevent the cascade of ageing-related concerns. We now have a growing body of research that only supports the positive links between fasting, disease prevention and longevity.

We now know that the signs of ageing we once accepted as inevitable are largely preventable. By integrating gentle fasting into your lifestyle, you can remain vibrant, active and youthful well into your later years. Would you give fasting a go if you knew you would feel lighter, happier, more focused and it wasn't too difficult?

Integrating fasting

Just as the body benefits from circadian rhythm, it also benefits from regular digestive rest. A one-day-a-week fast could be just the ticket to enable a sufficient cleanse to support the body's metabolism. Depending on your starting point, you could choose instead to do a day of eating lighter - reducing meal frequency, eating just fruit or a simple meal of *khichdi*, *see* pp. 136–7. This is often enough to give the digestive system a much-needed rest and a chance for the mind to gain clarity while benefiting from a mild caloric restriction.

The lunar connection

On the 11th day of both the waxing (*Śukla Pakṣa*) and waning (*Kṛṣṇa Pakṣa*) lunar phases comes *Ekādaśī*. This day is considered to be auspicious for fasting because it aligns with the gravitational pull of the moon. In the same way the tides of the ocean are impacted by the moon, so too is the movement of fluids in our body (we are 70 per cent water, after all). On the 11th day this pull is at a unique balance and provides us with an opportunity to naturally clear toxins and balance *doṣas*.

Many people feel naturally less hungry on this day - making the fast flow with ease. The fast gives space for *prāṇa* (life energy) to be directed away from digestion to deeper spiritual, emotional and physiological cleansing, thus cultivating *sattva* (clarity of mind), not to mention the positive impact on the gut microbiome and physical body. It is also believed that fasting on this day allows for *saṃskāras* (negative past impressions) to be gently cleared (*see* pillar 7).

Fasting for your body type

We're all unique and the way we fast and what works best comes down to listening to both good guidance and our genuine hunger cues. Here's how fasting can be tailored to your *prakṛti* - your unique constitution (for a refresher on *doṣas*, *see* pp. 37–43):

- ***Vāta*-dominant** folks are sensitive and prone to irregular digestion, so only benefit from gentle fasting. This means not skipping food entirely, but choosing light, easy-to-digest nourishment like warm broth, soups or a simple mono-diet of *khichdi* during the fasting window. Extended fasting can be overstimulating and destabilising for the *vāta* nervous system.
- ***Pittā*-dominant** individuals usually have a strong digestive fire, which means they may not be able to tolerate fasting. Therefore, it's best to avoid intense or prolonged fasting, so as not to aggravate *pittā* and become overheated or irritable. They do best with shorter fasts with cooling, hydrating support, such as herbal teas (like mint or fennel), diluted fruit juices, or coconut water during fasting hours. Avoiding spicy or acidic foods when reintroducing food after fasting is helpful for keeping *pittā* calm and balanced.
- ***Kapha*-dominant** people thrive on fasting! Their slower metabolism benefits from a more structured or intensive fast, such as eating fewer meals and choosing very light foods, like steamed and spiced veggies, herbal teas and broths during the fasting period, to counteract heaviness and lethargy.

Fasting in practice

Fasting doesn't need to be extreme to reap the benefits. Start small and build consistency, and over time it will become effortless. Here is what I suggest you try - you can tailor by factoring in your *prakṛti*.

Regular fasting

Aim for a minimum of 12 hours of fasting daily. This means that you will consume all calories within a 12-hour window, with your last meal at least three hours before bed. This could mean you finish your evening meal at 7 p.m. and don't eat anything until at least 7 a.m. the next day.

Why 12 hours? Well, it takes your body roughly 12 hours to use up the glucose supply stored in the liver. As these reserves deplete, your body's metabolism shift gears and may enter a mild state of what is known as ketosis – a metabolic state where your body primarily uses fat for fuel instead of carbohydrates. This simple change can lay the foundations for healthspan and longevity.

Unlike modern-day fasting that aims to lengthen the fasting window to induce metabolic effects, *Āyurvedic* fasting has a different intention. The aim is to restore digestion, not to maximise deprivation or be used as a routine practice in otherwise healthy individuals.

Fasting is a corrective tool used when digestion is impaired (*āma*), and it should naturally end once true hunger appears (*kṣudhā*) – a sign that *agni* is ready to welcome nourishment again. Signs that digestion is complete: the previous meal has no lingering tastes, belching is clear, the body feels light, energy and focus return, elimination is easy and genuine hunger appears naturally.

If fasting is prolonged, too intense or not suited to your *prakṛti* (constitution), it becomes depleting rather than beneficial – it can weaken *agni*, aggravate the *doṣas* and trigger imbalance. The body is no longer clearing *āma* but breaking down its own tissues (***dhātu-kṣaya***). For this reason, fasting is kept short and purposeful. Healthy fasting is marked by accurately recognising the return of healthy appetite and stable energy not by how long you can go without food.

Signs the body is being depleted rather than restored include light-headedness, dizziness, fatigue, bloating, feeling cold, irritability, anxiety and difficulty in sleeping.

Through trial, error and intuition, my daily fasting window ratio usually ranges between 16:8 or 17:7 hours per day, which seems to suit my *prakṛti* (predominantly *pittā* and *vāta*) and digestion, and in all honesty is not that hard for me. That feels like my limit, and I always listen to my body. Some days can be harder, and some days are just off-kilter, so if I don't hit 16 or 17 hours, I don't stress – sometimes hormones can often influence our fasting window – what's important is to not be fixated on the hours as a rigid 'goal'. In the *vāta* stage of life (55+), intense fasting is not recommended: a gentle *vāta*-aligned approach to eating, with simple, warm, grounding foods and regulated meal timings, is better suited.

Once you're comfortable with an overnight 12-hour fast, you may naturally be able tolerate a longer overnight gap of up to 16 hours, and this can be beneficial when it arises from a comfortable digestion and stable energy, not from pushing past hunger. For example, have dinner by 6 p.m. and eat your next meal at 10 a.m. the following day - try one or two days per week. This allows autophagy and *āma pācana* to be activated and work its magic.

Periodic fasting

The transition between seasons, known in *Āyurveda* as *ṛtu sandhi*, presents a natural window for a short, focused cleanse (or *Panchakarma* if needed). These few days are ideal for aligning the body with the rhythm of the new season ahead. Fasting or gentle *laṅghana* practices at this time help to release accumulated *āma* and restore digestive efficiency.

For example, early spring is the perfect time to clear out the *kapha* build-up from winter. As the weather warms, *kapha* naturally begins to liquefy and mobilise, which can lead to symptoms like mucous, allergies, dullness or weight gain if not properly cleared.

When we say things like '*kapha* build-up' or '*kapha* cleansing', we're referring to the heavy, moist, slow and sticky qualities that naturally accumulate during late winter and early spring. Even if you're not *kapha* by constitution, these qualities can affect anyone seasonally.

To support this transition, we turn to targeted *kapha*-reducing and *laṅghana* strategies like *dīpana-pācana*, seasonal fasting, cleansing herbs and a lightening diet. Think of it like a deep house clean! Even if you tidy daily, sometimes you need to open the windows, clear the corners and shake out what's been lingering. *Kapha* cleansing at winter's end is your body's version of spring cleaning, sweeping out heaviness so you feel lighter, clearer and ready for renewal. Autumn is another aligned opportunity for targeted cleansing, so you are more receptive to the deeper nourishment of winter.

Summary of fasting tips for pro-ageing

- Finish your evening meal three hours before bed, ideally around 6-7 p.m.
- Avoid snacking between meals. If you have an eight-hour eating window the objective is not to eat constantly but to have two nourishing meals and maybe one snack.

→

- Create an overnight fasting window of 12 hours, going up to 16 hours if your digestion allows – start where you feel comfortable.
- Warm clear liquids are encouraged during your fasting periods.
- If you feel unwell or extremely hungry, listen to your body and end the fast.
- Healthy fasting sounds like: 'I'm not feeling genuine hungry so my body is still processing and not ready to eat yet.'
- Unhealthy fasting sounds like: 'I'm genuinely hungry but I am overriding it to see how long I can go without eating.'

Important safety note: Before making significant changes to your eating patterns or if in any doubt, please consult a qualified healthcare professional. Fasting is not recommended for children, the elderly, or pregnant/breastfeeding/menstruating women. It is also contraindicated for anyone with a history of disordered eating, or those managing medical conditions, including type 1 diabetes, heart disease, or any chronic illness. Avoid fasting if you are underweight, unwell, deeply fatigued, taking medications that require food, or experiencing significant *vāta* imbalance. When in doubt, prioritise safety and choose the gentlest path for your body.

Eat less to live longer

How much we eat matters just as much as *what* and *when* we eat. While extreme diets may come and go, *Āyurveda* has always encouraged us to eat with awareness, in moderation and in tune with our body's natural rhythm.

Now research is showing that gentle calorie restriction, when done mindfully, may be one of the most powerful tools we have for longevity. But this should not mean extreme prolonged fasting, dieting or deprivation.

A common guideline for portion control is 'one ***añjali***' (the amount of food that fits in your cupped hands). If we ate according to this, we would stay in pretty good shape. *Āyurveda* also guides us to eat our meals only until we are three-quarters full in our stomach. These are the most accurate and personalised guidelines for the right amount of food in one meal.

The *Āyurvedic* approach is about alignment and sustainability. Simply cutting out unnecessary snacking and reducing portion size slightly can make all the difference. If you tend to indulge, a simple trick is to serve yourself as usual, then remove about 10–20 per cent of your meal or reduce your plate size. You don't need to put your body into a strong calorie deficit, just enough so that your body and digestion do not feel uncomfortable.

A word of caution for those in extended Indian families: there are always feeders urging you to have just one more roti or more sweets, piling food on your plate without asking and then telling you not to waste it. Learn to set healthy limits and boundaries with these well-meaning but unhealthy communal eating habits.

How to eat consciously

Most off-the-shelf diets fail because they focus on some kind of restrictions without considering the bigger picture of health. *Āyurveda* teaches us that the key to healthy ageing isn't about restrictions, rules and rigidity but about tuning into our body's natural intelligence.

For example, sitting cross-legged on the floor naturally restricts the stomach from overeating since the gentle bending back and forth to reach each morsel is a mechanism of communication between the brain and body to know when we've eaten enough. We also need to listen to other signals. When we feel a genuine hunger for the next meal, this is a sign that the previous meal has been fully digested. Eating before this will only contribute to indigestion and build-up of *āma* and in turn weaken the *agni*.

Your eating mindset

One idea from my early *Āyurvedic* training that never left me was that there is a trio of eating archetypes: the *rogi*, the *bhogi* and the *yogi*:

1. The ***rogi*** – is an indulgent eater who often eats three or more meals often at odd times, on the move, with a diet filled with →

heavy, ultra-processed, overly spicy, oily or excessively sweet foods. Digestion becomes sluggish. Energy is low, making it the perfect terrain for disease to fester. In fact, *rogi* translates as 'one who is diseased'.

2. The ***bhogi*** - is a sensual eater, enjoying gourmet, rich foods and yes, unable to resist that dessert you know you don't need. While this may be two organic, beautifully plated meals, it's often excessive and consumed more for pleasure than nourishment.
3. The ***yogi*** - is an intentional eater of simple, fresh, *sattvic* food, prepared and eaten consciously. The *yogi*'s often single meal honours the body, brings balance, presence and joy in nourishment. The body feels light, the mind is clear and digestion functions efficiently.

So, which of these did you resonate with? We tend to swing between them through life, but the goal is to move in the direction of the *yogi*.

Intuitive eating tips for pro-ageing

It's helpful to summarise here how *Āyurveda* can help you unlock your intuitive intelligence:

- Eat only when you are truly hungry.
- Avoid overeating - eat to only three-quarters of your stomach's capacity.
- Slow down the speed at which you eat (this prevents overeating).
- Maintain regular mealtimes. Eating at inconsistent times confuses digestion and disrupts circadian rhythms. Ideally:
    - Breakfast (light) between 7 and 9 a.m. (if hungry)
    - Lunch (main meal) between 12 and 2 p.m. when digestion is strongest
    - Dinner (lighter meal) by 5–7 p.m. to allow full digestion before sleep.
- Avoid snacking between meals. Allow three to six hours between meals for proper digestion.
- Eat warm, freshly prepared meals that support digestion, promote *ojas* (vital essence) and enhance *prāṇa* (life force).

- Eat in a calm, peaceful environment, engaging all your senses. Eating while distracted (TV, phone, work) reduces awareness and digestive efficiency.
- Chew food properly. Digestion begins in the mouth – chewing thoroughly sends signals to the stomach to release digestive enzymes. Try chewing each morsel 20–30 times.
- Eat according to your *prakṛti* (constitution):
    - Warm, moist, grounding foods for *vāta*
    - Cooling, hydrating and mildly spiced foods for *pittā*
    - Light, warm and well-spiced foods for *kapha*.
- Sip warm water before and after meals and avoid excessive fluids during meals. Cold drinks weaken *agni* and slow down digestion.
- Keep meals simple but include all six tastes (sweet, sour, salty, bitter, pungent and astringent – *see* p. 132).
- Avoid food incompatibilities. Mixing fruit with dairy or fish with milk, and hot food with cold food is considered incompatible as they disturb digestion and create toxins (*āma*).
- Finish your last meal three hours before sleep. Eating late at night disrupts digestion, the body's natural detoxification process, sleep and metabolism.
- Taking a moment to pause and offer gratitude for the food before starting the meal enhances digestion and mindfulness.

Water – your lifelong companion

Water (*jala*) doesn't simply hydrate us: it is a carrier of life, medicine and rejuvenation. As one of the five elements that form the human body, water plays a dual role of cleansing *and* nourishing. Its cool, smooth, soft qualities help pacify heat, dryness and roughness, especially in health conditions aggravated by imbalanced *vāta* and *pittā doṣas*, making it essential for pro-ageing. It also keeps the skin supple, the mind alert and the tissues juicy well into later life. It is, quite literally, a daily *rasāyana* of its own.

While modern health culture often fixates on hitting daily water targets like 'eight glasses a day', *Āyurveda* teaches us that water is *prāṇa* (life force) in a liquid form and that the focus should be quality, temperature and timing rather than quantity per se. In *Āyurveda*, warm or boiled water (*uṣṇodaka*) is considered light, subtle and more easily absorbed deep into the tissues. It kindles digestion, flushes toxins, soothes the channels and gently supports elimination. In contrast, large amounts of cold or treated water can weaken *agni*, hinder digestion and create sluggishness – something I've observed repeatedly in my clinic. Or how about sourcing your own fresh water from a nearby spring? (*see* Resources, p. 271 to find a local spring).

To support hydration and pro-ageing, sip warm water throughout the day, preferably between meals, rather than gulping large amounts in one go. A glass of warm water first thing in the morning acts as a gentle cleanser for the gut and energises the tissues. Avoid drinking too much just before, during or after meals, as it can dilute the strength of *agni*. Even better, infuse your water with herbs like cumin, coriander or fennel, or store in a silver vessel to calm excess heat in the body and support *ojas*. *How much water should I drink?* I hear you ask. My answer: thirst is your body's natural signal, so listen to it. Clear urine is the best sign you're well-hydrated.

Part 2

Seven pillars of pro-ageing

How to integrate the seven pillars of pro-ageing

Now that we have a clear understanding on the principles of *Āyurveda* and preparation for *rasāyana*, part 2 guides you to integrate and embody these insights.

The seven pillars of pro-ageing form a practical toolkit designed to strengthen your body, steady your mind, nourish your spirit and expand your sense of vitality. Each pillar offers simple yet impactful ways to create change, through reflections, rituals, nourishment and movement as we work through the layers of your being (*pañca kośa)*.

You can read this section from start to finish or dip into whichever pillar feels most urgent or relevant. It may feel natural to understand the cycles and rhythms of our lives first by reading pillar 1 and build momentum from there, but there is no right or wrong place to begin.

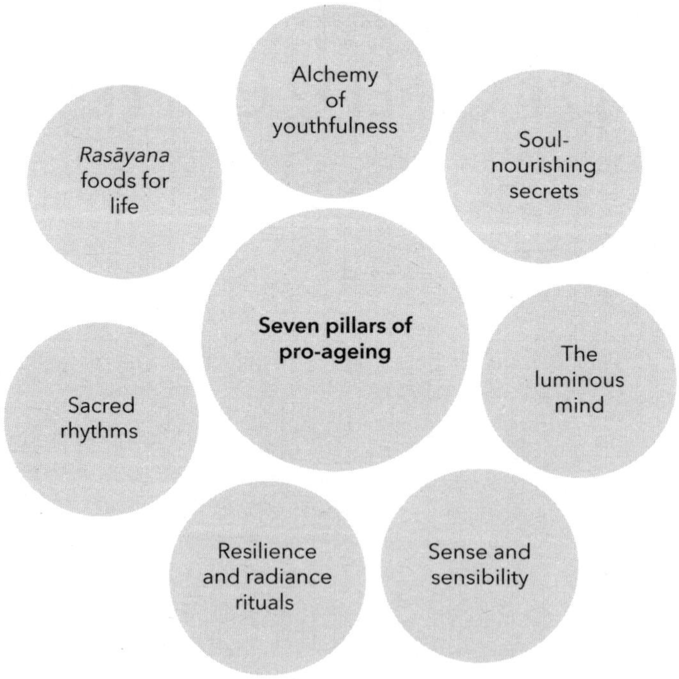

Figure 5.1 The seven *Āyurvedic* pillars of pro-ageing

We will explore:

- **Pillar 1: Sacred rhythms of self and nature** - An invitation to realign with nature's timing through daily and seasonal rhythms. Discover how better sleep, aligned mealtimes, personalised routines and rising early (***brahma muhūrta***) restores balance and vitality.
- **Pillar 2: *Rasāyana* food for life** - Explore how food is a powerful source of *rasāyana*. Through daily nourishment we can support lasting health and vitality through the six tastes, balanced use of fats and spices, and *ojas*-building meals that ground and uplift.
- **Pillar 3: Alchemy of youthfulness** - This pillar explores *dravya rasāyanas,* the rejuvenating herbs and formulas that are elixirs for strengthening body, mind and spirit, restoring balance and vitality from within.
- **Pillar 4: Resilience and radiance rituals** - Discover simple daily movement to build and maintain physical strength, rituals that nourish the skin and hair, while protecting yourself from the environmental stressors of modern life.
- **Pillar 5: The luminous mind** - Explore how to cultivate *sattva,* our inner state of clarity, balance and harmony. Here we learn how to nurture creativity, and calm the nervous system through breath, mantra, self-inquiry and silence.
- **Pillar 6: Sense and sensibility** - Learn daily rituals to care for your five senses, build emotional strength and nourish your 'social diet' through meaningful connection, stillness and emotional balance.
- **Pillar 7: Soul-nourishing secrets** - Rediscover the power of rituals, prayers, kindness and gentle practices that lighten the heart, release the past and restore a sense of meaning and peace.

Pillar 1

Sacred rhythms of self and nature

'Live in each season as it passes; breathe the air, drink the drink, taste the fruit, and resign yourself to the influence of the earth.'
Henry David Thorea, *Walden*

There was a time in my life when I was completely out of sync with myself, and with nature. A total prisoner to the work-hard, play-hard corporate world, because that's what I was conditioned to think 'discipline' looked like. I'd gulp down a carb-heavy breakfast on the go, squeeze in intense gym sessions at lunchtime, follow it with a cold 'healthy' salad, then soldier on through the afternoon with sugar hits. Evenings often ended in late dinners designed to impress, rather than nourish, paired with wines and other cold drinks. I'd wake up tired and groggy only to do it all over again and since everyone around me was doing the same, it was called 'normal' – it was 'just the culture'.

But when I quietened enough to hear the cues of my body's intelligence, I came to realise that health isn't found in following the herd mentality, fighting with willpower or following trends. It's rooted in the rhythm of nature. True vitality arises when we honour our *prakṛti* (unique constitution) and align with the cycles of the natural world: the rising and setting sun, the waxing and waning moon, the shifting of seasons. *Āyurveda* calls this *vihāra*, aligned lifestyle practices that preserve youthfulness and slow ageing.

In this pillar we will explore the powerful pro-ageing tools of:

- *Dinacaryā* (daily routine)
- ***Nidrā*** (sleep)
- *Ṛtucaryā* (seasonal rhythms).

Dinacaryā (daily routine)

'Yathā piṇḍe tathā brahmāṇḍe'

'As is the body (microcosm), so is the universe (macrocosm).'
Liṅga Purāṇa, 2.12.24

Like all living beings, we are a reflection of nature itself. When we live in sync with it, we return to our true self – which, as I've learned, is the crossroads between existing and thriving.

You've probably heard the phrase 'chasing the sun'. It evokes a longing for light, warmth, joy and freedom or perhaps simply making the most of our time. But from an *Āyurvedic* perspective, it's about something deeper: living in sync with the sun's rhythm – to rise with

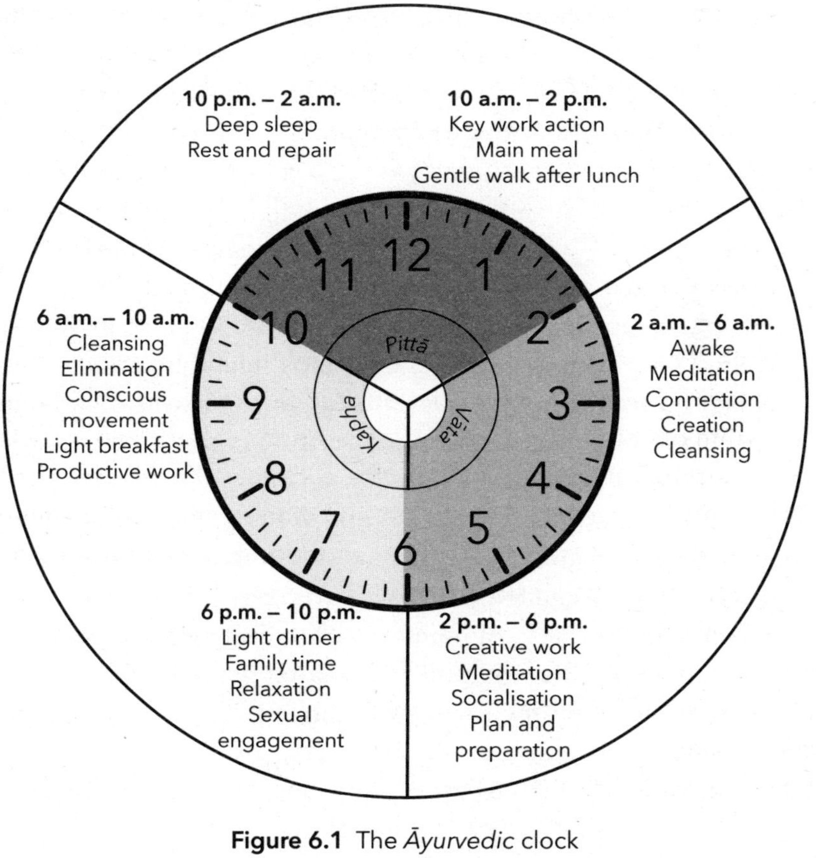

Figure 6.1 The *Āyurvedic* clock

it, flow with its energy and wind down as it sets. After all, the sun mirrors the fire (*agni*) within us that metabolises food, thoughts and experiences. It is deeply connected to our biological rhythms and the source of all life.

Today, 'circadian rhythm' has become a modern health buzzword. Coined by pioneer of chronobiology Franz Halberg in the 1950s, it refers to the body's internal 24-hour clock that governs sleep, digestion, hormones and more. Yet long before science mapped clock genes, *Āyurveda* had already recognised these energetic tides. Every cell in our body follows a rhythm that mirrors the cycle of nature.

The *doṣas*, the bio-energetic forces that govern our body, are the same energies that influence natures cycles – from day and night to the changing seasons. Understanding this pattern helps us to synchronise our digestion, sleep and energy to the rhythms of nature. By waking, eating, moving, cleansing, resting and sleeping in a timely way, we practise *dinacaryā*, the *Āyurvedic* art of living in harmony with the rhythm of the day.

The *Āyurvedic* clock (*see* Fig. 6.1) divides the day into three distinct time periods, each governed by a *doṣa* (*kapha*, *pittā* and *vāta*), which influence our energy, focus and metabolism as the day unfolds. Let's explore how we can align our activities with these energetic windows to support better health and vitality:

1. ***Kapha* time** (6–10 a.m. and 6–10 p.m.) – Mornings are ideal for cleansing rituals and invigorating movement to shake off the overnight stagnation and awaken the system. Sleeping in during this time amplifies sluggishness. Evenings should be about winding down with light meals, dim lighting, time with loved ones and soft self-care rituals. *Kapha* supports deep sleep, so getting to bed by 10 p.m. helps us tap into the zen energy of *kapha*.
2. ***Pittā* time** (10 a.m.–2 p.m. and 10 p.m.–2 a.m.) – During the day, this is our peak productivity window and ideal for decision-making, mentally challenging tasks and digesting our main meal when *agni* is strongest. At night, the body switches to internal housekeeping mode where the focus is on detoxification, repair and brain cleansing. If we're awake during this time, especially while on screens coupled with late-night munchies, we miss utilising the healing potential of sleep and may feel exhausted, irritable or restless.

3. ***Vāta* time** (2–6 a.m. and 2–6 p.m.) – In the early morning, rising before sunrise allows us to catch the stillness of *brahma muhūrta* (*see* pp. 102–3), a sacred time for meditation, reflection or breathwork. In the afternoon, *vāta* energy supports brainstorming, writing and creative tasks, but can easily turn into restlessness or distraction if not kept in check. *Vāta* naturally increases with age, so cultivating routine, warmth and inner calm becomes even more important.

There's something powerful about the transition periods of dawn and dusk. These are known in *Āyurveda* as *Sandhi Prakāśa*, the sacred junctions between light and dark, when nature shifts gears and the body becomes sensitive but equally responsive. The body's *doṣas* shift and circadian hormones reset. It's a perfect time to anchor in health-regulating practices such as breathing, meditating or simply pausing to reset your nervous system and calm the mind.

So, let's do that now. Take a moment to reflect:

- What do your energy levels feel like at different times of the day?
- How closely does your current routine align with the *Āyurvedic* rhythms above?
- Could you experiment by adjusting one or two habits this week to match the *Āyurvedic* clock?

Nidrā (sleep)

Of all the practices that support health and longevity, sleep might just be the most underestimated. In *Āyurveda*, *nidrā* (natural, restorative sleep) is considered one of the three anchors of life, alongside diet (*āhāra*) and balanced sexual energy (*brahmacharya*). Without sleep, the body and mind simply cannot repair, restore or rejuvenate. It is the exact reason we tend to sleep more when we are sick.

Let's explore what disrupts deep rest, why the timing of sleep matters as much as the duration, and how rising with the sun can transform your energy. You'll also find a simple 'sleep hygiene checklist' here to help you reclaim truly restful nights.

The silent healer

I didn't always value and honour sleep the way I do now. In my 20s, I believed pushing through exhaustion was a badge of honour. But the more I listened to my body, the more I realised deep, restorative sleep isn't a luxury: it's non-negotiable for vitality, especially as we mature.

With age, *vāta doṣa* (air and space) naturally increases, bringing its qualities of lightness and irregularity into the body. This shows up as lighter and more erratic sleep. If we ignore signs of imbalance, it can gradually deplete *ojas* (vital essence). Sleep disturbances may seem minor, but over time, it can mute our mental clarity, drain energy and affect mood.

The energy of *kapha* (water and earth) is naturally slow, heavy and grounding – the very qualities that help us fall into a deep, restful sleep. This state of stillness supports the body's repair processes, strengthens the immune system and helps replenish *ojas*. During sleep, the brain also clears out waste and toxins (a concept now echoed in neuroscience as the glymphatic system).

Good sleep is more than simply resting each night – it's a process of deep healing. It's how we stay mentally clear, emotionally balanced and physically resilient. I've felt first-hand how delicate this balance can be. During perimenopause, subtle hormonal shifts began to affect my sleep; I would wake up wired at 3 a.m. or feel exhausted yet restless at night. It was a stark reminder that even small internal shifts can create a ripple effect, tipping us into a cycle of poor sleep, low energy and heightened stress. In a world where we glorify hustle, I'd argue that the most radical act of self-care might simply be going to bed on time.

Rhythm and blues: sleeping in sync with nature's rhythms

Our bodies are wired for rhythm: day and night, light and dark, season to season. And sleep resides at the heart of this rhythm.

Modern-day sleep experts suggest that seven to eight hours of daily sleep is optimal for most of us but according to *Āyurveda* and from my experience, it's not just about how many hours we get, but more about when and how deeply we rest. Eight hours of sleep between midnight and 8 a.m. isn't the same as sleeping between 10 p.m. and 6 a.m. Sleep timing strongly affects our metabolic health. I've observed so many clients thrive, not by adding more hours but by simply adjusting their sleep schedule – a real game changer.

We're designed to rise and rest in synchrony with the sun. When the sun goes down, your eyes send signals to the pineal gland to release melatonin, one of our most vital hormones that helps regulate our sleep-wake cycle. But nowadays, we live in a constant glare of blue light – from indoor lighting, TVs, laptops and phones – and our bodies simply aren't built for it. Energy-efficient LEDs are among the worst offenders. In the daytime, a dose of blue light is helpful as it creates alertness and lifts mood but at night, it tells the brain to stay awake when we should be winding down. The more blue light we absorb at night, the more we disrupt the delicate communication between our eyes, brain and gut, which regulates digestion, mood and circadian rhythm. Over time, this disconnection accelerates ageing.

In contrast, cortisol, our natural 'get up and go' hormone, rises with the morning sun, working in opposition to melatonin, which peaks at night. When these rhythms are disturbed, we wake up tired and wired, only to then struggle to sleep when it's finally time to rest.

Melatonin supplements are everywhere now, but like most quick fixes, the results rarely last. I prefer rituals over remedial hacks. Having said that, herbal allies like *aśvagandhā*, valerian root, chamomile, lemon verbena or a pinch of nutmeg in warm milk can gently work wonders with a little consistency.

But here's what's often missed – rising with the sun and exposing our eyes to natural morning light helps reset our circadian clock, boosting serotonin by day and melatonin by night. Vedic scriptures have long encouraged the practice of honouring and gazing at the sun in the morning as a way to reconnect with the source of all life. Early-morning sun exposure strengthens *agni*, balances hormones and improves the quality of sleep, energy, mood and alertness, especially when done within an hour of sunrise. It's for the same reasons we practise ***Sūrya Namaskāra*** (sun salutations) at this time.

In the evenings, I like to keep things soft and mellow: dim lighting only, switching to a red bulb in the bedroom before sleep, and candlelight in the bathroom. Red light is gentler on the nervous system and is the least disruptive on melatonin production. Maybe there's even something symbolic in it too: red for the root ***chakra*** (the first of seven energy vortices along the spine that influence physical and emotional well-being) is for safety and grounding us back into the body.

Going to bed by 10 p.m. aligns us with the body's natural cycles and allows us to tap into *pittā*'s repair window between 10 p.m. and 2 a.m. when both cellular detox and the glymphatic system are most active as we sleep.

Top tips for optimal sleep

Something many people don't realise is the impact of late-night eating on sleep. When digestion is still active at bedtime, the body diverts energy away from the healing that is meant to be happening. Light evening meals and regular sleep–wake patterns help prevent build-up of *āma* (toxins), protect *ojas* (immunity) and are pro-ageing.

Rhythm matters, but rigidity can be harmful. What we want is to maintain a fluid and flexible discipline. I always tell my clients to think like animals. They don't need alarm clocks; they instinctively follow the light. I do the same. In the UK, the robins and blackbirds are my natural morning call. Are you ready to use nature as your alarm clock?

Instead of a morning alarm clock, I now use a 'bedtime alarm clock' as a gentle reminder to unplug and begin to wind down. I give myself at least 45 minutes, ideally an hour, to transition – just like our ancestors would have done.

Late nights are often romanticised, especially when we're younger. I've even heard people say 'I'll sleep when I'm dead' but sleep deprivation accelerates ageing and increases risk of chronic disease. Just one week of poor sleep can throw your body into imbalance and mimic the effects of chronic illnesses like diabetes or heart disease. And while there's a myth that we need less sleep as we age, the truth is, we need more grounding, not less. So, let's not take sleep lightly – literally!

The golden hour invitation: *brahma muhūrta*

Do you want to be among the first to catch the sun's earliest rays, soaking in light that lifts your energy, sparks creativity and supports longevity?

Yogis (established practitioners of yoga) understood that the key to youthfulness and clarity lies in waking during *brahma muhūrta*, the sacred window about 1.5 hours before sunrise (typically between →

3.30 and 5.30 a.m., depending on location). It's a time of deep stillness, when the world feels paused and the veil between the physical and spiritual realms is thinnest. In the *Ashtāṅga Hṛdaya*, it's said that rising at this time supports longevity, health and success in all areas of life.

Brahma muhūrta literally means 'the creator's time', an ideal moment for inner work, self-care, spiritual practice, intuitive downloads and creative flow. About seven years ago, my body began waking naturally at this hour. At first, I resisted it, thinking it was disrupting my sleep, but it became a doorway to deeper alignment. The more I honoured this rhythm, the more clarity and connection followed.

Many of the most grounded and successful people I know or have read about, rise early – not from pressure, but from knowing this is when inspiration truly flows. It's not about perfection but about consistently creating more healthful habits.

Pro-ageing exercise: Honouring the rising sun

This is a quick but powerful way to wake up your entire body, boost your mood, feel grounded and ready for the day ahead.

How to practise:

1. Step outside and look at the rising sun within an hour of sunrise, when the light is soft, ideally before 7 a.m.
2. Gaze gently for a few seconds or up to two minutes without sunglasses but don't strain, then close your eyes and feel the warmth.
3. Optionally, add a mantra like *'Om Suryaya Namaha'* (pronounced *Om Soor-yaa-ya Na-ma-huh*), translated as 'I bow down to the sun god', chanting aloud or silently with devotion.
4. Let the sound rise from your belly and move with your breath.
5. Or simply breathe with gratitude.

Sleep hygiene checklist

Good-quality sleep can be nurtured through daily habits. Here's a simple checklist to guide you:

- Our core body temperature drops around bedtime so if you are up watching TV and you reach for that blanket, take it as a sign that it's time to go to sleep. One of my favourite evening rituals is a warm shower before bed to help me unwind mentally and emotionally, and the subtle drop in temperature afterwards seems to ease me into deeper sleep.
- Create a quiet, dark space that mimics the *kuti praveśikā* model (rejuvenation therapy in isolation) by using blackout blinds, eye masks, earplugs or soft background sounds like natural white noise (river stream, rain, crackling fire).
- Fresh air and calming essential oils like lavender, chamomile or vetiver can also help prepare the mind for sleep.
- Aim to go to bed by 10 p.m. and wake up before sunrise (*brahma muhūrta*) for maximum rejuvenation.
- Avoid anything stimulating and allow time to unwind with evening rituals such as oil massage (***abhyanga***), breathwork, meditation, journalling, a warm bath or drinking warm milk with spices (e.g. nutmeg, cardamom, cinnamon, turmeric or *aśvagandhā*) to promote restful sleep.
- Eat a light plant-based evening meal – nothing heavy at least three hours before sleeping. If you really need something, have a hot spiced milk drink (builds *ojas*).
- Avoid heavy, spicy or acidic meals before bedtime, as they disrupt digestion and sleep quality; we all know how this feels!
- Gentle stretch and strength exercises are OK but nothing too vigorous.
- Avoid blue light in the evening and choose dim, candle or red lighting.
- Exercise during the morning – kapha time is ideal.
- Get green exposure by walking in nature during the day to ground yourself.
- Reset your circadian patterns with some early-morning sun exposure (*see* the rising sun practice and *brahma muhūrta* above).

- Write down your worries, ideas and to-do list. If it is out of your mind and on the paper, then you can rest better.

Ṛtucaryā: sync with the seasonal rhythms

Each season encourages us to adjust our routines especially around sleep, movement, and what, when and how we eat – we're now tapping into our 'infradian' rhythms. Our bodies intuitively want to flow with these shifts, but modern life drowns out our ability to fully tune into these signals. *Ṛtucaryā* teaches the wisdom of seasonal living to help us align and flow with these natural transitions.

Winter

We naturally sleep longer in winter, when nights are longer and *kapha* energy encourages deep rest and repair. Digestion and physical energy are at their strongest at this time and winter is the body's prime season to build resilience, replenish our deepest reserves and build *ojas*. I see winter as the time for nourishing *rasāyana* foods (like nuts, seeds, root veggies, healthy fats and warm drinks – more on this in pillar 2) and deep rest, but balanced with strengthening movement, warm baths, steam baths, saunas and exposure to morning sunlight.

Spring

In spring, the *kapha* stagnation of winter begins to melt and lighten. It should feel easier to wake up earlier and feel more refreshed. Spring is the ideal time for cleansing, with lighter, spiced foods (soups, dals, steamed greens, herbal teas) and movement that energises without exhausting us. Easy wins are brisk walks, dry body brushing (***garśana***) and uplifting yoga.

Summer

Summer, ruled by *pittā*, brings longer days, shorter nights and a natural rise in dispersed internal heat. This season calls for foods that keep you cool energetically such as fresh greens, cucumber, mint, juicy fruits and tender coconut, along with gentler movement such as swimming, moon salutations or early-morning walks before the sun intensifies. Evening wind-down rituals become essential to soothe the system and balance the inner fire.

Autumn

The dry, light and erratic *vāta* energy dominates autumn. Sleep often becomes lighter too, especially with age. This is the season to focus on warm, grounding meals like soups, root vegetables and healthy fats, and oil massages as well as slow, stabilising movement like restorative yoga or walks in nature.

Pro-ageing exercise: seasonal awareness

Take a few minutes to reflect on your answers to these prompts:

1. What season am I currently in (based on where you live)?
2. How does my body and mind respond to this season (energy levels, digestion, sleep, mood, cravings)?
3. What small adjustments can I make in my food, movement or sleep routine to align more with the season's qualities (e.g. eating lighter in spring, going to bed earlier in winter, consuming warming foods in autumn)?

Pillar 2

Rasāyana food for life

'From food all beings are born; by food they live; into food they enter – for food is the eldest of beings.'

Taittirīya Upaniṣad

As the ancient *Āyurvedic* proverb wisely puts it: 'When diet is wrong, medicine is of no use. When diet is correct, medicine is of no need.' And really, you only have to pause long enough after a meal to notice how food makes you feel to realise the truth in that.

In chapter 5, we laid the foundations that help you to cleanse your system and rekindle your digestive fire. Pillar 1 then explored how you can align with the rhythms of nature. In pillar 2, we turn to what sustains it all: *āhāra* (food).

Āyurveda sees food not just as fuel, but as nutritional medicine, capable of either building vitality or slowly depleting it. Now that your digestion is reset and your body more attuned, you're ready to receive the full nourishment food can offer.

In this pillar, we'll look at:

- Our food landscape today
- Why food is considered the foundation of *rasāyana*
- How to eat in ways that nourish and rejuvenate the mind and body with everyday foods
- The wisdom of intuitive eating through taste (*rāsa*) and how they restore balance
- The role of spices and oils in amplifying vital energy (*ojas*)
- The importance of antioxidant and inflammation-reducing foods in modern life
- A treasure chest of ***medhya rasāyana*** (foods that support the brain and steady the emotions)
- Six magic recipes to invite *rasāyana* into your kitchen.

Food as medicine

न चाहारसमं किञ्चिद्भैषज्यमुपलभ्यते ।

na cāhārasamaṃ kiñcid bhaiṣajyam upalabhyate |

'There is no medicine comparable to food.'

Kāśyapa Saṃhitā, Khilasthāna 4.5

In *Āyurveda*, *āhāra* is integral to healing and the primary source of nourishment for our tissues. *Āhāra rasāyana* is the art of using food as medicine to rejuvenate both body and mind. When we eat in alignment with our unique constitution (*prakṛti*), honouring seasonal and circadian rhythms, local climate and the strength of our digestive fire (*agni*), *āhāra* becomes our most potent pro-ageing flex.

Food is the foundation of health both for the body and the microbiome, but only when it is fully digested and absorbed (*see* chapters 3 and 5). We often say 'We are what we eat' but more accurately, we become what we absorb (nutrients) *and* don't absorb (toxins). If the body doesn't recognise or process what we consume, our microbiome gets disturbed, leading to dysbiosis, and our tissues are left undernourished. Instead of fuelling tissue vitality, we create biological confusion, accumulate toxins, trigger inflammation and accelerate ageing.

Five thousand years ago, there were no protein bars or potato chip packets; *āhāra rasāyana* referred to foods that were simple, seasonal and packed with *prāṇa* (lifeforce energy). Though our diets have changed dramatically, the principles remain timeless - making this wisdom more relevant than ever. Before diving into the specifics, though, let's pause to look at our modern food landscape.

The food landscape today

Our current health crisis is two-fold: overfed and undernourished. The problem isn't a lack of calories but too many choices, many of which don't serve us, leading to overconsumption and with it, a surge in lifestyle-related disorders.

Ironically, the way our bodies were designed to thrive – with simple, nourishing meals at the right times – now gets labelled a 'diet'. In truth, healthy eating is as much about what we include as what we leave out. But packaged foods claiming to be 'fortified' with nutrients doesn't mean they qualify as real nourishment. Real foods don't need an ingredients label; they carry their nutrients naturally.

In just half a century, calorie intake in the UK and USA has surged, with over 60 per cent of daily calories now coming from ultra-processed foods – that's up from an estimated less than 5 per cent two centuries ago. In the USA, the average adult now eats around 2,200 calories per day, and highly processed foods make up nearly two-thirds of what children and teens consume. This pattern fuels obesity, diabetes and heart disease, with poor diet contributing to nearly 700,000 deaths each year in the USA alone. Large population studies show that those who consumed the most ultra-processed foods are dramatically more likely to die early compared to those who eat the least. If we don't change our eating habits, these numbers will only rise, making food choices a matter of life and death.

We're filling our bellies but not necessarily feeding our bodies. Today's packaged foods are energy-dense but nutrient-poor – loaded with refined sugars, emulsifiers, hydrogenated fats and synthetic additives, while lacking fibre, micronutrients and, most importantly, *prāṇa*. *Āyurveda* calls these *asātmya āhāra* – foods that don't suit your body or mind. Over time, *asātmya āhāra* weaken the tissues, compromise *ojas* and strain the immune system.

The modern misunderstanding of food

It seems to me that we are living in a strange nutritional paradox. We can easily get caught up in the online fearmongering around natural foods presented as harmful. Staple foods like rice, oats, fruit, ghee and other natural ingredients are sometimes scrutinised for containing harmful compounds based on single metric data, insinuating that they don't deserve space on our plate. This approach often misses the big picture view and notably, NHS guidelines and credible nutritionists support these staples as vital sources of nutrients.

For example: **basmati rice** is demonised for spiking blood sugar – yet it's a low-medium GI, an easily digestible staple especially when old grains are eaten in moderation and paired with ghee, dal or vegetables to create balance.

Lentils and beans are often avoided because they contain lectins, deemed as 'toxic anti-nutrients', but proper soaking, sprouting and cooking well (as we've done for generations) negates this and makes them deeply *sattvic* and protein-rich.

Oats, nuts and seeds are called out for 'blocking mineral absorption' due to the phytic acid, but when soaked – as per *Āyurvedic* tradition, they're antioxidant and support long-term tissue health.

Meanwhile, we rarely question the health washing of zero-calorie sweeteners, synthetic protein powders, processed foods and are even suitably impressed by lab-made foods.

The message here is to be mindful how you outsource your food choices to trends, extremes or social media 'experts' and rather understand the context, preparation and pairing of food. It's time to reclaim agency over our dietary choices. *No* food from nature is inherently good or bad. What we've lost is the ability to distinguish between real and processed foods and understanding how natural foods can be transformed in both good *and* bad ways through processing.

Rasāyana foods for pro-ageing

Longevity isn't found by cutting out big food groups in our diet while simultaneously popping supplements or nutritional powders – it's built through honest nourishment. The whole is always greater than the sum of the parts. The synergy of nature's intelligence matters. A clean, seasonal *sattvic* diet rich in *prāṇa-* and *ojas*-building foods *is* the ultimate pro-ageing medicine.

Rasāyana foods are daily nourishment that don't simply replenish our immediate energy needs; they are life-enhancing foods that sustain healthy metabolism, restore strength, build resilience, uplift immunity (*Vyādhi-kṣamatva*) and sharpen our mental clarity. Collectively, *rasāyana* foods are rejuvenating, functional and they slow ageing and degeneration.

A *rasāyana*-rich diet works best when the body is receptive, free from *āma* (toxins), with a digestive system that's firing on all cylinders to transform food into high-quality *rasa*. This subsequently nourishes all the other *dhātus* (tissues) and ultimately creates *ojas* – the foundation of vitality. When *ojas is* abundant, we feel energised and emotionally steady, and it gives us that unmistakable *joie de vivre*. When *ojas* is depleted (*ojakṣaya*), it can bring fatigue, restlessness, lowered immunity and a lack of joy can set in.

A food could be considered *rasāyana* in functional terms, if it:

- Prevents formation of *āma* - reducing metabolic stress and oxidation
- Reduces inflammation - keeping body pathways open (*srotas*) and flowing
- Regenerates tissues and enhances strength (***bṛṃhaṇa***) - supporting growth, repair and recovery from depletion
- Is compatible (*sātmya*) - (*sattvic* and *prāna*-rich) and easy to assimilate by the body
- Promotes *ojas* - strengthening immunity, emotional steadiness, mental clarity and vitality
- Delays ageing (*vayasthāpana*) and supports longevity (*āyuhprada*).

Building and Balancing *Rasāyana* foods

When it comes to diet for longevity and vitality, *rasāyana* refers to the functional nature of food: it can have a primarily 'building' effect (*bṛṃhaṇa,* nourishing and *ojas*-promoting) or a 'balancing' effect (supporting metabolism and rejuvenation). *Rasāyana* foods are generally *sātmya* when they are compatible, easily assimilated by the person and supporting the body over time. It is worth noting that the same food can behave differently depending on the context of the person's constitution, digestion, presence of *ama* (toxins) or body strength.

Building *rasāyana* foods tend to focus on providing quality (and quantity) of nourishment required to support, strengthen and develop healthy *rasa* (nutritive plasma) and enhance *ojas* (vital essence). Foods with a building effect are essentially warm, moist, grounding meals that include root vegetables, grains, dairy, healthy fats and well-cooked proteins (legumes and animal). Of these, *Āyurveda* highlights some key *ojas*-promoting foods which we will explore later.

Balancing *rasāyana* foods, on the other hand, tend to support and optimise the body's natural metabolism, tissue renewal and function, helping to reduce excess and keep the system clear. Foods that have a balancing *rasāyana* effect include leafy greens, fibrous vegetables, lighter fruits and spices with bitter, pungent or astringent tastes. These are usually rich in antioxidants and anti-inflammatory by nature. Either way, we need a personalised blend of both building *and* balancing foods for pro-ageing.

As we age, *vāta* (the principle of movement and air) naturally increases, bringing more dryness, depletion and gradual tissue loss. Modern culture often tends to amplify this, with an obsession over cleansing, extreme fasting and cutting back large food groups - all very lightening (*laṅghana)* by nature and aggravating for *vāta*. While useful and necessary at times, in excess - especially as we mature into the *vāta* stage of life - prolonged and excessive *laṅghana* can be highly depleting, especially if metabolism is already strained.

From our 40s onwards it becomes especially important to lean into more *ojas*-promoting nourishment that maintains resilience, stability and vitality for the long run. What are you 'adding back in' to nourish your tissues and spirit? Add more variety, more colour, more plants, more spices. You may notice your body feels grounded, agile, calmer and more at ease.

So, what is a nourishing diet for longevity and vitality? Think of it as a sliding scale based on your age, *agni* strength, health issues and the season - for example, favour more building and *ojas*-promoting foods during *vāta* phases (autumn, winter and older age) and include more or less balancing *rasāyana* foods accordingly throughout. Balance for a healthy 45-year-old female with stable *agni*, after having cleared *āma* through *laṅghana* for example, may look like this:

- 60–70% building *rasāyana* foods - helping replenish, nourish and feed the tissues, maintain strength and muscle mass. Here the focus is on increasing *dhātu* quality and building *ojas*. *See* Table 7.1 overleaf.
- 30–40% balancing *rasāyana* foods - helping to keep digestion strong, toxins at bay and channels clear, keeps a check on *kapha* stagnation and prevents metabolic disorders linked to ageing (antioxidant rich and anti-inflammatory foods). *See* Table 7.2, p. 114.

The best way to tell if your ratio is working for you is by revisiting the vitality and *agni* checklists on pp. 49 and 73–4.

Table 7.1 below gives examples of **building** *rasāyana* foods (for tissue quality and growth) and Table 7.2 gives examples of **balancing** *rasāyana* foods (anti-inflammatory and antioxidant rich) to include, so you can start to create a healthy balance. Some foods can be *both* building and balancing – so the trick is to not be too rigidly attached to food lists.

Food group	Building foods for tissue quality and growth
Grains	Basmati rice, red rice, brown rice, whole wheat, buckwheat, oats, semolina, quinoa, spelt, barley, sorghum (*jowar*), finger millet (*ragi*), foxtail millet, amaranth
Dairy	Warm cow's milk, ghee, fresh paneer, lassi (sweet or mildly spiced), fresh full-fat yoghurt (in moderation), goat cheese
Legumes	Green gram (whole and split mung beans), black gram (whole and split *urad dal*), pigeon pea (*toor dal*), red and green lentils. Adzuki, black-eye beans, lima, pinto beans. Well-cooked chickpeas or kidney beans with ghee
Fruits	Bananas, mangoes, dates, raisins, figs, avocados, cherries, stewed apples and pears, *amalaki* (Indian gooseberry), melons, pomegranate, papaya, jackfruit, persimmons, peaches, cooked green plantain
Vegetables	Root vegetables (sweet potatoes, carrots, beets, yam, taro, cassava, jicama), squashes (pumpkin, ash gourd, bottle gourd, summer or acorn squash, asparagus, peas)
Fats and oils	Ghee, sesame oil, coconut oil, almond oil, small amounts of olive oil
Nuts and seeds	Almonds, cashews, walnuts, pine nuts, pistachios, soaked sesame seeds, pumpkin seeds, black sesame seeds, poppy seeds, flax seeds, chia seeds, tahini, almond butter
Spices and condiments	Mild warming spices like cardamom, fennel, saffron, cinnamon (used in nourishing dishes), tamarind
Animal products	Organic chicken, beef, pork, duck, lamb, bone broths, fresh river fish, eggs, salmon, sardines
Sweeteners	Jaggery, maple syrup, honey (raw, used properly – *see* p. 123), dates, molasses

Table 7.1 Building *rasāyana* foods

Food group	Balancing foods with anti-inflammatory and antioxidant properties
Fruits	Berries (blueberries, strawberries, raspberries, cranberries), cherries, *amalaki*, pomegranate, pineapple, papaya, oranges, stewed apples, grapes, mangoes, figs, dates
Nuts and seeds	Almonds, walnuts, pistachios, hazelnuts, pecans, chia seeds, flax seeds, sesame seeds, pumpkin seeds, sunflower seeds, hemp seeds
Oils and fats	Ghee – in *pitta*-related inflammation and in absence of *āma*, extra virgin olive oil (EVOO), extra virgin coconut oil (EVCO), flaxseed oil, hemp seed oil, mustard oil, avocado and avocado oil, oily fish and fish oils
Vegetables	Leafy greens (spinach, kale, Swiss chard, collard greens, mustard greens, rocket), cruciferous vegetables (broccoli, Brussels sprouts, cauliflower, cabbage, kohlrabi), bitter gourd (*karela*), drumstick leaves (*moringa*), courgette, pumpkin, ash gourd, beetroot, carrots, sweet potatoes, asparagus, okra, mushrooms (shiitake, maitake), tomatoes, onions, garlic
Whole grains	*Śāli* rice (unpolished white rice), barley (*yava*), quinoa, farro, oats, millets (*rajgira, bajra, jowar*), brown or red rice, buckwheat, rye
Legumes	Mung beans (highly recommended in *Āyurveda*), red lentils, chickpeas, black beans, peas, split peas, split pigeon peas (*toor dal*), cooked bean sprouts
Culinary spices and herbs	Turmeric, ginger, cinnamon, coriander, cumin, black pepper (enhances curcumin absorption), cayenne, carom seeds (*ajwain*), mustard seeds, holy basil (*tulasī*), garlic, fenugreek, fennel seeds, cardamom, cloves, mint, rosemary, thyme, sage, raw honey
Beverages	*Takra* (*Āyurvedic* buttermilk), green tea, matcha tea, herbal teas (***triphala*** tea, *tulasī* tea, ginger tea, chamomile tea)

Table 7.2 Balancing *rasāyana* foods

Your anti-inflammatory and antioxidant toolkit

Chronic inflammation is undeniably the key trigger of many health conditions, from heart disease to arthritis. One of the simplest, most direct ways to calm it is through what's on our plate – through balancing *rasāyana* foods.

At the epicentre is a colourful mix of anti-inflammatory and antioxidant-rich foods that not only help combat chronic inflammation but support tissue repair, immunity and graceful ageing. Antioxidants are firefighters in our body, protecting our tissues from the daily wear and tear of life. Carotenoids such as beta-carotene in carrots and lutein in leafy greens, and polyphenols found in berries, pomegranates, green tea and a little coffee all help defend against oxidative stress. Vitamins C and E, found in *amalaki* (Indian gooseberry), citrus and almonds, work well as our body's security guards. Minerals like zinc in seeds and magnesium in soaked almonds act like our internal ambulance service, actively repairing cells. Other powerful defenders policing our body include glutathione (whose production in the body is supported by sulphur-rich foods like garlic and cruciferous veggies) and Coenzyme Q10 (in organic meats, fish and whole grains). Together, these nutrients act as a defence team, keeping inflammation and oxidative stress at bay, while protecting *ojas*, and preventing *dhātu* degeneration.

What's fascinating is how modern nutritional science is beginning to echo these ancient principles. The spotlight on metabolic flexibility, nutrient density, dietary diversity and microbiome health maps beautifully on to this framework of building and balancing foods. It's a reminder that the body doesn't thrive on extremes, but on rhythm and personalised balance; exactly the wisdom of the *āhāra rasāyana*.

Ojas-promoting foods for pro-ageing

Ojas is formed when we nourish the body with building *rasāyana* foods while our *agni* (metabolic fire) is stable; refer to p. 34 for a reminder of this process. If our *agni* is weak or foods are not nourishing (*asātmya*), we are likely to develop *āma*, not *ojas*.

Interestingly, many *ojas*-promoting foods are naturally rich in minerals like potassium, which is vital for cellular energy and balance. Simple, daily foods like bananas, spinach, sweet potatoes, berries and avocados build sustainable vitality and a varied diet keeps our inner ecosystem alive and thriving.

One key example of a complete *ojas*-supporting, tissue-nourishing food is a warm bowl of spiced rice pudding. This seemingly simple dish of rice, milk, ghee, spices, jaggery and dates is a wholesome hug for the cells and the soul.

Key *ojas*-promoting foods

We want our daily diet to build resilience for our future self. This brings us to some of the most time-honoured restorative treasures in *Āyurveda* – or '*Āyurvedic* superfoods' as I like to call them.

Milk and dairy

Now, this may ruffle a few feathers, especially in today's climate where dairy is often avoided for ethical, environmental or digestive reasons, but in *Āyurveda*, cow's milk is considered a wholesome food and one of the most potent *rasāyanas*. We are referring here to fresh, raw, unhomogenised and boiled A2 cow's milk – milk that contains only the A2 beta-casein protein, believed to be easier to digest and less inflammatory than the common A1 casein milk. When it's organic, ethically sourced, fresh and prepared properly (*see* the tip overleaf), milk builds *ojas*, nourishes all tissues (*dhātus*) and supports longevity, calming both body and mind.

Āyurvedic texts describe milk as ***soma***-rich (cooling and rejuvenating), grounding and deeply *sattvic* (pure, mind-calming and life-supporting). It's especially beneficial during the evening hours, when spiced and taken warm to enhance digestion. A bedtime cup of warm milk with nutmeg or turmeric is both comforting and medicinal for the nervous system.

Goat's milk is another option that is lighter and easier to digest than cow's milk, making it a good choice for those with slower digestion. Sheep and buffalo milk are also referenced in classical texts, used therapeutically according to constitution and condition.

Pro-ageing tip: how to use milk

To use milk as *rasāyana*, always boil it; never drink it cold from the fridge. Cold milk is challenging for digestion as the proteins are tightly packed and can weaken *agni*. The heating process loosens the proteins, making the milk lighter and easier to digest. Combine it with spices like turmeric, saffron, ginger, nutmeg or cardamom to enhance digestibility.

Sip slowly and avoid combining with sour, salty, fermented foods or fruits as they are considered incompatible food combinations. Known as *viruddha āhāra*, certain food with opposite qualities that digest at different rates can cause putrefaction, weaken digestion and block the body channels. Have you noticing how some foods like fruit and yoghurt smoothies can sit heavy?

Nuts and seeds

Rich in healthy fats and oils, nuts and seeds provide essential nourishment that strengthens and restores the body's tissues. Almonds support brain and skin health, while walnuts, pecans and pistachios are deeply nourishing. Sesame seeds are especially valued in *Āyurveda* for building *ojas* and supporting bone, skin, hair and reproductive health. Black sesame seeds are mineral-rich and rejuvenating while white seeds are lighter and easier on digestion. Other *ojas*-promoting seeds include pomegranate and pumpkin. Soaked nuts and ground seeds enhance nutrient bioavailability.

Ghee and other fats

Traditional cultured ghee made from cow's milk into yoghurt, then churned into cultured butter and heated to form ghee is often called 'liquid gold' in *Āyurveda*. It is the most celebrated *rasāyana* fat with its sweet, unctuous, cooling and regenerative qualities, what's more, it contains butyric acid, fat-soluble vitamins (A, D, E, K) and omega fatty acids. When *agni* is strong, used in appropriate amounts, suited to your constitution – ghee is great dietary ingredient. Ghee nourishes the body, is easy on digestion, supports immunity (*ojas*) and cognitive clarity (*sattva*). In the modern context, although, ghee is 60–65% saturated fat, it is composed mainly of short-chain fatty acids (SCFA), which can be a digestible source of energy – unlike other sources of saturated fats such as meat fats and palm oils. The issue we face today is that with an already highly processed and fatty diet the benefits of ghee may easily be outweighed.

Ghee is generally used as a cooking fat in small amounts. It is suitable for high temperature cooking due to its high smoke point, making it less likely to oxidise or produce free radicals when heated. Traditional ghee is said to support vision, improve voice tone, restore physical strength, mental steadiness, improve complexion and preserve age. It is, quite simply, one of the finest *rasāyana*s for stabilising, preventing degeneration and is pro-ageing.

But ghee's benefits go beyond the kitchen. In *pañcakarma*, for example, specially prepared medicated ghee is used to cleanse *and* nourish the tissues at the same time. It softens and mobilises toxins (*āma* & vitiated *doṣas*), ready for elimination while simultaneously soothing and lubricating the tissues in your body so they can function better – genius!

A word of caution: Ghee should be consumed in moderation. Avoid ghee if you have high *āma* (caused by heavy or processed foods), low *agni*, excess *kapha* in the body, during respiratory infections, or if you have a fatty liver or cardiovascular risk factors. Consult a healthcare provider about appropriate amounts for your individual health needs. Modern shop-bought ghee may still be fine in cooking but may not carry the same medicinal value as traditional cultured ghee.

Healthy fats are a key component of *rasāyana* foods, so I want to dive a little deeper into the subject of oils and fats for pro-ageing as well as explore 'good' v 'bad' fats.

Well-oiled for well-being

Hydration isn't just about drinking water; it's also about keeping the body well-lubricated with healthy fats, especially as we move into the *vāta* stage of life (*see* p. 41).

Āyurveda has always seen fats as more than a macronutrient: they're medicine for the body and mind. If your mind feels foggy, your joints creaky, your skin dry or your mood a little off, it's a sign that it might be time to oil your inner channels. Both *Āyurvedic* wisdom and modern science agree that healthy fats nourish every cell and are instrumental to healthy ageing.

If the idea of adding more fats to your diet makes you worry about calories or cholesterol, let me put your mind at ease. Fats have long been misunderstood, demonised as culprits for weight gain and heart disease. In fact, they're essential, particularly as we age.

Our brains are nearly 60 per cent fat by dry weight, and every single cell in the body relies on lipids for structure, communication and repair. In fact, studies show how omega-3 fatty acids reduce inflammation, support heart health and are vital for brain health. And here's a fun fact: Inuit populations, with their high-fat diets, rarely suffer from heart disease.

Did you know that some of the most vital nutrients in your food, such as vitamins A, D, E, and K, are fat-soluble? That means they need dietary fat to be properly absorbed and delivered to your tissues. Without enough good fat, those expensive supplements might not be doing all that much!

One of the primary drivers of chronic conditions such as arthritis, anxiety, depression and heart disease is inflammation and the right fats are an anti-inflammatory powerhouse. In *Āyurveda*, good fats pacify *vāta*, soothe the tissues and support mental calm. Extra virgin olive oil heals the blood–brain barrier and provides neuroprotection, with studies showing 28 per cent lower dementia mortality.

Good v bad fats

Let's think of your body like a car. It needs fuel, water and oil to run but if you put in the wrong fuel or oil, it means the car may move but may not drive smoothly. Well, this is the same for our mind/body. Fats influence the body differently, depending on their type. They can either support longevity or accelerate wear and tear.

Healthy fats like omega-3 and omega-6 fatty acids are essential for energy, hormonal balance, brain function, cellular repair and the absorption of vital nutrients. Omega-3s (including ALA, EPA, DHA and DPA; don't worry about the full names!) are found in foods like flaxseeds, walnuts, chia, cold-water fish and algae. They act like internal coolants, reducing inflammation, stabilising mood and keeping joints supple and skin hydrated. Healthy fats are both *bṛṃhaṇa*- and *ojas*-promoting.

Omega-6 fats (such as linoleic acid) can also be beneficial when balanced with omega-3s, especially when sourced from whole foods like sesame seeds, sunflower seeds, pumpkin seeds and avocados. The problem is that most modern diets are overloaded with omega-6s from processed oils, skewing the balance and instead, promoting inflammation and causing havoc for our mitochondria (cellular powerhouses). Fats from margarine, fried or baked snacks (trans and hydrogenated fats) are best kept to a minimum due to links with heart disease and other metabolic conditions. Cold-pressed oils preserve *prāna* and vital nutrients while commercial refined seed oils due to their lack of *prāna* and *tamasic* nature are best limited to small amounts when your diet also includes plenty of whole foods and omega-3s.

Table 7.3 shows some beneficial fats to include in a pro-ageing diet.

Fats to include	Benefits
Cultured ghee	Sacred and *sattvic rasāyana* in *Āyurveda*. Rich in omega-9s and butyric acid. Aids digestion, nourishes the brain, pacifies *vāta*, builds *ojas*.
Cold-water fish (salmon, mackerel, sardines)	High in EPA and DHA. Supports heart and brain health.
Sesame oil	Warming, strengthening, *sattvic*. Excellent for *abhyanga* (oil massage) in *vāta* season.
Flaxseeds, chia seeds, walnuts	Excellent plant-based omega-3 sources. Reduces inflammation, supports cardiovascular and skin health.
Avocado	Nourishing, hydrating and rich in potassium and fibre. Supports skin, joint and hormone health.
Coconut oil	A stable cooking fat; cooling and especially suitable for *pittā* types.
Extra virgin olive oil (EVOO)	Anti-inflammatory. Rich in polyphenols. Supports cardiovascular health.

Table 7.3 Fats to include

Now we understand the nuances with fat. Let's continue with our *ojas*-building food exploration.

Seasonal vegetables

Organic seasonal vegetables are nature's most intuitive *rasāyana* offerings, both *sattvic* and *prāna* rich. When we eat in alignment with the seasons, we support the body's natural cycles of cleansing, rebuilding and maintenance. These foods give us exactly *what* we need, *when* we need it.

In spring (*laṅghana* season), bitter and astringent vegetables like spinach, spring greens and drumstick leaves (*Moringa oleifera*) help clear accumulated *kapha* and support gentle detoxification. Their lightness and bitterness stimulate digestion and support the liver.

Traditional Indian vegetables such as ash gourd (*kuṣmāṇḍa*/winter melon) – a revered classical *rasāyana* – along with white gourd and Indian spinach are cooling, hydrating and restorative, especially for *pittā* and in warmer seasons. Many of these are rich in trace minerals and antioxidants, offering subtle *rasāyana* effects when well-cooked (*see* the pro-ageing tip below) and eaten regularly.

As the weather cools into autumn and winter (*bṛṃhaṇa* season), nature gives us a harvest of more grounding and nourishing vegetables such as carrots, beets, pumpkin and sweet potatoes. Naturally sweet and warming, they balance *vāta*, strengthen the tissues and help maintain stability and resilience.

Pro-ageing tip: how to cook vegetables well

Favour cooked over raw vegetables as they are gentler on digestion – breaking down fibres, increasing nutrient bioavailability and supporting *agni*. Light steaming or sautéing with ghee and spices like cumin or ginger enhances their digestibility and energetic potency. Always opt to eat freshly cooked when it comes to veggies to ensure maximum *prāna*.

Fresh, ripe, sweet fruits

Fresh, ripe, organic, seasonal (and in an ideal world – local) fruits are an important part of a *rasāyana* diet, provided they are sweet, soft, easy to digest and eaten alone. *Amalaki* (Indian gooseberry) stands out as one of *Āyurveda's* most revered classical *rasāyanas*, a powerhouse of natural vitamin C, which rejuvenates the tissues and supports immunity (*see* pp. 144–5). *Dādimā* (pomegranate) is celebrated in the texts as a *rasāyana* for its deeply hydrating, vitality-enhancing and digestion-supporting qualities. It nourishes the skin, balances all three *doṣas* and acts as a tonic for the heart – benefits that are now recognised equally in modern science. Grapes are cooling and support eye health, vocal strength and hydration.

Bananas, though heavy, are strengthening, aphrodisiac and supportive of both cardiac and muscular function. Mangoes are similarly nourishing and support the heart, enhance the senses and build tissues. Coconuts are both cooling and restorative, acting as tonics for the brain, heart and urinary system. Avocados, rich in healthy fats, help repair and rebuild tissues, making them an excellent modern-day *rasāyana*. The intelligence of nature still never ceases to amaze me!

Dried fruits

Dates, soaked raisins, figs, prunes and – my recent obsession – sun-dried apricots are energy-dense, strengthen tissues and build *ojas*.

Dates, particularly Medjool dates, are highly valued among *rasāyana* foods. Rich in nutrients and deeply anabolic, dates build strength, energy and resilience. They are a perfect example of nature's nourishing sweetness that supports both physical and mental well-being.

Their unique nutritional profile makes dates exceptionally *balya* (strength-promoting). Packed with fibre, antioxidants and micronutrients like potassium, magnesium and trace minerals, they naturally replenish the body and help fight oxidative stress. Unlike refined sugars, the natural sweetness of dates is bound to fibre, slowing absorption and stabilising blood sugar levels, for sustained energy without the 'crash'.

By neutralising reactive oxygen species (ROS) in the body – natural by-products of metabolism that accelerate cellular ageing and inflammation – dates support tissue repair, cellular vitality and immunity.

Try this: Pair one to two Medjool dates with a teaspoon of almond butter, soaked almonds or walnuts, or even a little ghee and cinnamon, for a satisfying, deeply nourishing snack.

Consuming one to two Medjool dates (or any dates, though Medjool are best) a day can be a simple yet profound way to support energy, promote tissue health and cultivate vitality. They are a perfect snack for those recovering from illness or experiencing fatigue, as they provide immediate yet sustained nourishment.

Raw honey

Raw honey (*madhu*) is a *laṅghana* food but a potent ingredient when used correctly - raw, unheated and in moderation. Naturally antibacterial, antioxidant, prebiotic and nutrient-rich, it supports gut health, balances blood sugar levels and enhances the absorption of other *rasāyana* substances (*yogavāhi*).

In Ikaria, Greece, a designated blue zones region, many elders take honey daily (consumed as medicine). A teaspoon a day is sufficient to reap its *rasāyana* benefits. It is good for the eyes, voice, complexion, intellect and vitality and is an aphrodisiac, while helping to balance obesity and mental fatigue.

Whole grains and legumes

Red rice (*śāli*, particularly *śāstika śāli*) is highly regarded in *Āyurveda* as a *classical rasāyana grain* due to its light and strengthening properties and easy digestibility. It replenishes the tissues, supports longevity and promotes *ojas*.

Ancient grains like oats, barley, spelt and wheat (*godhūma*) are grounding and tissue-building, ideal for a *rasāyana*-supportive diet. Barley is praised for toning the voice and supporting healthy fat metabolism. Finger millet (*ragi*) - rich in antioxidants, amino acids, calcium and iron - supports sleep, metabolic balance, builds strength and stamina and gets a big pro-ageing thumbs up, especially when cooked with ghee. Among legumes, mung beans (*mudga*) are considered a *bṛṃhaṇa* staple that is light, nourishing and easy to digest, making them suitable for all *doshas*. Black gram (*māṣa*) is heavy and deeply strengthening, nourishing muscles, fat and reproductive tissue and building resilience.

Is wheat the culprit of our gut health issues?

Wheat has been under scrutiny for quite some time, with many choosing a 'gluten-free' diet due to the digestive discomfort it brings (different to Coeliac disease). No surprise as our modern diet is increasingly processed and laced with pesticides. While pesticides are designed to kill pests, they can also disrupt soil microbial communities and may indirectly alter our gut microbiota. Our microbiome is inherently designed to help us digest harder-to-handle foods like wheat, legumes, nuts and grains. When these microbes die out, our ability to digest these 'tough' foods also breaks down – we blame the food and call it an intolerance instead of realising that our *agni* is impaired (it's the same story with antibiotics). Here's the irony – simply removing challenging foods like wheat could weaken gut immunity further.

You may be surprised to know that *Āyurveda* praises *godhūma* (wheat) as nourishing and strength-giving. Studies show that whole, unprocessed wheat is linked with better metabolic health, while refined wheat is linked with higher rates of metabolic syndrome. It's clear that the issue is less about wheat itself and more about what we've done to our food, coupled with the state of our digestion. Small amounts of harder-to-digest foods act as hormesis – a gentle stress that strengthens our digestive and immune systems over time.

Perhaps it's time to train our gut the way we do our muscles and opt for breads made the old-fashioned way? Stone milled wholewheat, water, salt, slowly fermented, made into fresh *rotis*.

Pro-ageing tip: switch up your grains seasonally

Variety is key. Rotate grains and legumes seasonally: lighter ones in spring/summer (mung beans), heavier ones in winter (black gram).

Meat, meat soups and bone broth (for specific needs)

Many are surprised to find meat mentioned in *Āyurveda*, but classical texts such as the *Suśruta Saṃhitā* describe the therapeutic use of a wide range of animal meats, including chicken, goat, pork, beef, buffalo, fish and partridge along with many more obscure species that are not commonly seen today. While a plant-rich diet is generally encouraged, *Āyurveda* recognises that in times of illness, recovery or extreme tissue depletion, meat-based broths and soups can play a valuable restorative role. As always, the emphasis is on appropriate use, guided by the individual's condition, strength and digestive capacity.

Most meats are considered nourishing, strengthening and even aphrodisiac in quality. As *Āyurveda* teaches, *like increases like*, so consuming muscle tissue can help rebuild muscle mass when it's lost. These foods provide concentrated nourishment when used appropriately. That said, recent trends favouring high-protein and low-carb diets often go too far in the opposite direction. As always, balance is key and the context, constitution and condition best guide our choices.

Takra – the original probiotic

There's a huge trend towards taking over-the-counter probiotics and digestive enzymes, but I believe these solutions are not truly holistic or sustainable in the long run. Sometimes the simplest remedies carry the deepest healing.

Thousands of years ago, *Āyurveda* already had an answer in *takra*. Revered as the 'divine healer' for its *ojas*-protecting qualities, *takra* is *Āyurvedic* buttermilk - a simple, refreshing yoghurt-based drink designed to restore a healthy gut microbiome. The *Bhāvaprakāśa* text praised *takra* for its ability to prevent disease and maintain digestive strength when consumed daily.

Unlike shop-bought buttermilk, which is often processed and high in fat, homemade *takra* is a light and easy-to-digest *rasāyana* drink that restores digestive balance, reduces bloating and acidity, and supports long-term health and vitality. By stimulating *agni* (digestive fire), *takra* helps prevent the build-up of *āma* (toxins) and supports the formation of *ojas*. In fact, it may well be one of *Āyurveda's* best-kept digestive secrets.

Takra is made by churning natural yoghurt with water (1:4 ratio) to separate the fat. Spices like cumin, ginger, coriander and rock salt are added to enhance its digestibility and *doṣa*-balancing effects, particularly pacifying for *vāta*.

Thanks to its natural probiotic properties, *takra* enriches the gut flora, improves nutrient absorption and supports immunity. Quite possibly the first-known probiotic, this *sattvic* yet powerful drink calms the nervous system and nourishes all seven *dhātus* (tissues), helping to relieve fatigue and mental fog.

Traditional *takra*

In my Gujarati family, we call it *chaas* – a staple, always lovingly made with fresh homemade yoghurt.

Serves 1

Ingredients:

- 60ml (¼ cup) fresh natural yoghurt
- 250ml (1 cup) boiled and then cooled water
- ¼ tsp roasted ground cumin
- pinch of rock salt (Himalayan preferred)
- Optional: roasted ground carom, fresh coriander, black pepper, dry ginger

Method:

1. Blend the yoghurt and water until smooth.
2. Skim off any froth.
3. Add the cumin, salt and any optional spices, then stir and enjoy at room temperature.

Pro-ageing tip: when to drink *takra*

Drink *takra* around midday or after lunch, when digestive fire is strongest, to get the greatest *rasāyana* benefit.

→

Foods that support the brain

Herbs, foods and spices that enhance intellect, focus and memory are known in *Āyurveda* as *medhya rasāyana* – think of them as nature's nootropics. Certain foods can help nourish, support and protect the brain against cognitive decline as well as help reduce inflammation and protect against oxidative stress as we age. Let's look at some modern-day foods that are *medhya* in effect – you will notice some of the usual suspects.

- **Almonds** – The brain champions: rich in healthy fats and vitamin E, they protect against oxidative stress and support neural communication. Soak overnight and remove the skin for better nutrient absorption.
- **Walnuts** – High in omega-3s that boost mental sharpness and reduce inflammation when soaked. (Their brain-like shape is no coincidence!)
- **Sesame, sunflower and pumpkin seeds** – Provide plant-based zinc that support nerve tissue and strengthen brain function, especially if soaked or ground.
- **Ghee (cultured)** – Nourishes brain tissue and enhances nutrient absorption. A classic *medhya rasāyana*.
- **Cow's milk** (organic A2) – Deeply nourishes tissues and build *ojas*, supports sleep and protects against stress.
- **Dates and soaked raisins** – Replenishing for excess *vāta*, fatigue, stress by acting as a nervine tonic.
- **Fresh coconut (and coconut oil)** – Coconut is cooling, unctuous and nourishing in nature which can help balance *Vāta* and *Pittā* – *Vāta* being prone to dryness and depletion, and *Pittā* to heat and inflammation.
- **Dark leafy greens** (e.g. spinach, kale, broccoli) – Packed with folate and antioxidants to help prevent inflammation and cognitive decline.
- **Whole grains** (e.g. quinoa, finger millet (*ragi*), cooked *śāli* rice) – Indirectly sustain steady mental energy and help regulate blood sugar.
- **Ash and bottle gourd** – Light, cooling and nourishing. Protective for brain and mental clarity.
- **Turmeric** – Its active compound curcumin is anti-inflammatory and neuroprotective.

→

- ***Amalaki* (Indian gooseberry)** - Strengthens the nervous system and enhances clarity.
- ***Āyurvedic* herbs** - *Aśvagandhā, brahmi, gotu kola* and *tulasī* are known to enhance memory, focus and calm (*see* pillar 3).
- **Blueberries, salmon, eggs, EVOO, avocado, pomegranate, honey, dark chocolate and green tea** - Antioxidant-rich and support cognitive function by protecting the brain from oxidative stress and inflammation.

Culinary *rasāyana* spices for life

Spices are more than flavour enhancers for livening up your cooking. They're potent plant medicines and have supported digestion, immunity and longevity for thousands of years. Derived from the roots, bark, buds, seeds, fruits and leaves of plants, typically dried and used in small amounts.

Modern science is now on board with what *Āyurveda* has always advocated - that every pinch of spice can transform both flavour *and* function. Spices are rich in polyphenols, a broad group of naturally occurring plant compounds with powerful antioxidant and anti-inflammatory effects. These compounds belong to a diverse family of phytochemicals that help plants defend themselves and, remarkably, offer similar protective benefits to us. In spices, these polyphenols are highly concentrated, giving even the smallest pinch the potential to reduce oxidative stress, protect cells and support long-term vitality.

While my ancestors loved spices for their ability to make food taste better, they also recognised their ability to both preserve food in the absence of refrigeration as well as the healing impact through spicing synergy (*prabhāva*).

Rasāyana-friendly spices

- **Turmeric**:* Revered for its anti-inflammatory, antioxidant and immune-enhancing properties. Turmeric shines in soups, curries, dals, teas or golden milk.
- **Ginger**:* A digestive powerhouse that stimulates circulation and clears stagnation. Perfect in teas, curries, or grated fresh into dressings and broths.

- **Saffron**:* A brain tonic that enhances cognition, reduces stress and supports reproductive health.
- **Cinnamon* and cardamom**:* Both support digestion and respiratory health. Cinnamon adds warmth to porridges, while cardamom balances sweetness in desserts and milk-based drinks.
- **Cumin, coriander and black pepper**:* Foundational spices in *Āyurvedic* cooking. They aid digestion, reduce bloating and improve the bioavailability of other nutrients. Black pepper especially enhances the absorption of turmeric's active compound, curcumin, improving its bioavailability.
- **Nutmeg and mace**: Calming, grounding and slightly sedative. Traditionally added to warm milk at night to support restful sleep and calm a busy mind.
- ***Ajwain*, black cumin seeds and rock salt**: Time-honoured digestive aids traditionally used after meals to ease gas and heaviness. Use in spice blends or digestive teas to balance *vāta* and *kapha*.
- **Cloves**: Antiseptic, analgesic and warming. Use whole in dals and spice blends or ground in chai masala to clear respiratory congestion and aid oral health.
- **Garlic**:* Garlic is a cardiac tonic, supports cholesterol regulation and enhances memory, perception, complexion and male vitality. Used sautéed in ghee or oil (to temper its sharpness); it acts as a rejuvenator (*rasāyana*) that supports strength, throat health and stability in ageing.
- **Fennel seeds**: Sweet, cooling and digestive. Excellent for post-meal digestion as a tea or chewed whole, to refresh the breath and soothe the stomach and reduce gas and bloating.

*classical *rasāyana* supportive spice

Behind the spice scene

Spices trigger a mild stress response in the body, a process called *hormesis*. Although it may sound negative, this effect actually boosts resilience and helps cell repair. Their polyphenols and essential oils neutralise free radicals, regulating inflammation, reducing oxidative stress and promote tissue repair.

Simple ways to use spices daily:

1. **Start small**: Add one spice to an existing dish, such as cumin to roasted vegetables or cinnamon to porridge.
2. **Snacks**: Sprinkle garam masala on popcorn, enjoy a nut-stuffed Medjool date dusted with cinnamon or cardamom.
3. **Drinks**: Try turmeric or saffron-infused (golden) milk, ginger tea or spiced chai for a warming beverage with health benefits.
4. **Dips and dressings**: Add garlic, cumin and coriander to Greek yoghurt for a flavourful dip.
5. **Experiment**: Use ready spice blends like garam masala, *panch phoran, bāhārat* or ras el hanout as an easy way to elevate everyday recipes if you're new to spicing. Soon you'll be spicing up everything!

Spices are a simple and gentle way to weave *rasāyana*-supporting ingredients into your meals. By enhancing flavour and function, they bring your meals to life while supporting digestion, immunity and vitality. Start by exploring your spice box and let these tiny but mighty ingredients work their magic in your kitchen!

How to integrate *rasāyana* foods

Think of *rasāyana* foods as your dietary foundation, not an add-on. You don't need to overhaul your diet, just gradually adjust it with more wholesome foods. Aim to include at least one or two *ojas*-promoting foods daily, such as warm milk, ghee, soaked dates, mung dal or cooked root vegetables. Prepare them simply, with spices that support your *agni*.

Follow the seasonal cues. In colder months, choose grounding dishes like spiced porridge, warm milk tonics or *khichdi*. In spring, turn to lighter options like seasonal greens, fruits, *amalaki* (Indian gooseberry) juice or gentle herbal teas with *tulasī* and liquorice. In summer, cooling foods like dates, mango, ash gourd or tender coconut balance heat and maintain hydration. In autumn, stay calm and steady with warm, lightly spiced dishes, root veggies, sweet fruits and a touch of ghee.

Above all, *rasāyana* is a way of life, not a short-term diet and consistency wins every time. One truly nourishing meal, eaten mindfully, can have more impact than a supplement, thanks to the synergy of nature's intelligence, *prāṇa* and your awareness.

Start by upgrading what's already on your plate. Could breakfast become a *rasāyana* ritual with porridge made with ghee, cardamom, dates and almonds? These foods are timeless staples that build *rasa* and resilience for the years to come.

The role of the six tastes

In *Āyurveda*, digestion begins with taste – incidentally also known as *rasa*. To nourish our seven *dhātus* (sustaining body tissues) and maintain *doṣa* balance, we want our meals to include six tastes: sweet, sour, salty, bitter, pungent and astringent.

A meal with all six tastes in the right proportions for your constitution and current state of health satisfies the palate and ensures that all our nutritional needs are met, helping to build *ojas* and expand our healthspan. These six tastes support healthy digestion, stimulate metabolism and influence everything from tissue repair to emotional well-being. To me, this simple and intuitive approach to health by balancing taste is deeply sophisticated and truly unparalleled.

Often containing hints of other tastes, *ojas*-building *rasāyana* foods are primarily sweet in nature, but to state the obvious, this isn't a green light for cakes, pastries and confectionery. We're talking about the natural sweetness of nourishing foods like milk, grains, fruits and roots that are grounding, build *rasa*, strengthen the tissues, balance *vāta* and bring contentment to the mind and body. Listen up, carb fearers: a lack of sweet taste can leave your tissues undernourished, your energy low and, ironically, trigger sugar cravings (and not for the good kind, either!), a sign of *ojas* depletion. The takeaway? Not all carbs are the enemy. The culprits of chronic conditions such as weight gain, inflammation and diabetes are excessive refined carbohydrates and sugars.

Equally important, though less quantity is required, is the bitter taste – found in leafy greens and many spices such as turmeric. Bitter is *laṅghana* (lightening) to the body, clearing metabolic waste and balancing *pittā*. Without enough bitterness, digestion slows down and *āma* builds, but too much can be depleting.

Your taste receptors have a dual role, to both experience flavour and fire signals to your stomach to release enzymes and hormones that activate the digestive process by identifying its taste. Each taste plays a different physiological role, so by including all six, you lay the foundations for healthy nutrient absorption and assimilation.

We want the food in our diet to truly count, not just to fill a hole, especially if we intend to eat a little less (*see* pp. 88–91).

Table 7.4 outlines how the six tastes shape nourishment and support graceful ageing.

Taste	Primary action for pro-ageing	Food examples
Sweet (***madhura***)	Nourishes, strengthens and builds tissues and *ojas* (life essence). Calms nerves. Essential for vitality and longevity. Excess causes lethargy and excess weight.	Root vegetables, sweet fruits, whole grains, milk, dates, almonds
Sour (***amla***)	Stimulates digestion, improves appetite, supports absorption, maintains mineral balance. Excess leads to acidity and inflammation.	Lemons, vinegar, tamarind, fermented foods, yoghurt, pickles
Salty (***lavana***)	Enhances taste, stimulates digestion, maintains electrolyte balance, supports hydration. Excess accelerates ageing and increases *pittā* and *kapha*.	Rock salt, sea salt, seaweed, anchovies, olives
Bitter (***tikta***)	Purifies tissues and channels, reduces *āma* (toxins), mucous and inflammation. Excess weakens tissues, appetite and aggravates *vāta*.	Bitter melon, aloe vera, turmeric, dark chocolate, dandelion greens
Pungent (***kaṭu***)	Stimulates digestion, metabolism, circulation and clears toxins. Supports mental clarity. Excess leads to dryness, tissue depletion and *pittā* imbalance.	Black pepper, chillies, cloves, garlic, mustard, rocket
Astringent (***kaṣāya***)	Absorbs excess moisture, tightens and stabilises tissues, reduces inflammation and excess fat. Excess causes dryness, constipation and anxiety.	Pomegranate, green tea, green vegetables, artichoke, chickpeas

Table 7.4 The six tastes and their effects

Let's recap on the most important message for a *rasāyana* diet: nourishment is not static. We need to stay constantly adaptable to the seasons, the climate, our age and our *prakṛti*. Our diet must be both functional and contextual or in other words, aligned with nature *and* your nature.

Six magic *ojas*-promoting recipes

These recipes are just a taste of what's possible when you start to view food as a source of long-term vitality, not merely short-term sustenance. I appreciate this is not an extensive recipe collection, but I wanted to include a few nourishing, *ojas*-promoting sweet, savoury and sippable recipes that showcase how *rasāyana* ingredients can be integrated into your daily life. I encourage you to experiment with seasonal produce, trusted *Āyurvedic* staples, adaptogenic (stress-regulating) herbs and *rasāyana*-enhancing spices in your own kitchen. Let these recipes be a template you can evolve and adapt.

Bedtime *ojas* milk

Infused with ancient *rasāyana* herbs and warming spices, this tonic is more than a nightcap, it's a gentle invitation to sink into stillness, restore your *ojas* and nourish the body's subtle energies as you drift towards sleep.

Serves 1

Ingredients:

- 250ml (1 cup) organic A2 whole milk or almond milk
- ¼ tsp ghee
- 1 tsp ground or finely chopped almonds
- 1 tsp finely chopped pistachios
- ¼ tsp *aśvagandhā* powder
- pinch of saffron threads
- ⅛ tsp ground cardamom
- Generous pinch of nutmeg
- ½ tsp jaggery (or honey – only after milk cools slightly) →

Method:

1. Gently warm the milk in a small pan over low heat. Do not allow it to boil vigorously.
2. Stir in the ghee, almonds, pistachios, *aśvagandhā*, saffron, cardamom and nutmeg.
3. Simmer on a low heat for 5–7 minutes, allowing the herbs and spices to infuse.
4. Add the jaggery, if using, then blend with a stick blender (optional) for a smooth, creamy texture.
5. If you're using honey, let the milk cool slightly before stirring it in. Serve warm.

Śatāvarī-rose *soma* milk

Śatāvarī is one of *Āyurveda's* premier *rasāyana* herbs (*see also* p. 143), revered for supporting hormonal health, emotional resilience and deep rejuvenation. Paired with rose, cardamom and nourishing milk, this *soma* milk builds *ojas*, softens the heart and calms the nervous system, making it a perfect evening ritual, especially for females.

Serves 1

Ingredients:

- 250ml (1 cup) organic A2 cow's milk or almond milk
- ¼ tsp ghee or almond oil
- ½ tsp *śatāvarī* powder
- ⅛ tsp ground cardamom
- 1 tsp rose powder (food grade)
- ½ tsp jaggery or honey
- dried rose petals, to garnish (optional)

Method:

1. Gently warm the milk and ghee (or almond oil) in a small pan over low heat. Avoid boiling it vigorously.
2. Stir in the *śatāvarī* powder, cardamom, rose powder and jaggery if using. Whisk gently until mixed well.
3. Simmer for 2–3 minutes on low heat to allow the herbs to infuse.

➔

4. Turn off the heat and stir gently.
5. Pour into your favourite cup. If using honey, add when slightly cooled.
6. Garnish with a few dried rose petals for beauty and softness, if you like.

Amaranth energy bites

If you know me, you will know I cannot go a day without chocolate. So, these gorgeous bites are my heavenly but healthy indulgence – packed with yummy *rasāyana* ingredients to get me through the autumn and winter months. They are so easy to make and popping amaranth is fun. They are gluten-free, dairy-free, refined sugar-free and 100 per cent vegan.

Makes around 36 bites

Ingredients:

- 30g (1½ cups) pre-popped amaranth
- 100g (1 cup) unsweetened shredded or desiccated coconut
- 320g (2 cups) mixed seeds (sunflower, chia, sesame, pumpkin, linseed, flax)
- 100g (1 cup) roughly chopped nuts (pistachios, almonds, walnuts)
- 50g (1 cup) dried sour cherries or cranberries
- ½ tsp ground cinnamon
- ½ tsp ground cardamom
- 2 tsp *aśvagandhā* and/or *śatāvarī* powder (optional)
- 170g (1 cup) almond butter
- 330g (1 cup) date syrup
- 2 tsp vanilla extract
- 160g (1 cup) 100% unsweetened chocolate, roughly chopped

Method:

1. In a large bowl, combine the popped amaranth, coconut, seeds, nuts, cherries or cranberries, spices and *aśvagandhā* and/or *śatāvarī* powder, if using. Stir well to mix.

→

2. In a small pan, gently melt the almond butter and date syrup over low heat for about 2 minutes, until blended. Turn off the heat and let it cool slightly (it should stay liquid). Stir in the vanilla extract.
3. Pour the wet mixture over the dry ingredients. Mix thoroughly to coat everything evenly.
4. Add the chopped chocolate and mix again, ensuring it is evenly distributed.
5. Line a 35 x 35cm/14 x 14in square baking tray with parchment paper. Transfer the mixture on to the tray and press down firmly, smoothing the top with a metal spoon or spatula.
6. Refrigerate for at least 2 hours, until fully set.
7. Once set, lift the paper on to a wooden board. Using a sharp knife, slice the mixture into equal-sized squares or bars.
8. Store in an airtight container. I like to use a traditional steel *dubba* (tiffin box) and keep it in the fridge or a cool, dry cupboard for up to one month (if they last that long!).

Variations: You can experiment with this dish very easily. Try substituting different nuts, seeds, cranberries or goji berries. Substitute popped quinoa for amaranth. You can also add maca root or lion's mane mushroom powder as alternatives to the *aśvagandhā* and/or *śatāvarī* powder.

The ultimate Āyurvedic *khichdi*

Serves 3-4

Ingredients:

- 100g (½ cup) split green or yellow mung dal
- 50g (¼ cup) white basmati rice
- 3 tsp ghee
- 2 tsp cumin (+ optional whole spices: ½ tsp coriander, fennel, fenugreek)
- ½ tsp turmeric
- 1 medium chopped onion
- 1½ tsp rock salt (to taste)
- 2 tsp fresh ginger
- 450g (3 cups) chopped vegetables of your choice (1cm/1/2in size) e.g. carrots, green beans, sweet potato
- 750ml (3 cups) hot water (may need to add more)

→

- 50g (1 packed cup) of chopped spinach
- Lemon juice to taste and chopped coriander, to garnish
- ¼ tsp black pepper
- 1 bay leaf (optional)

Method:

1. Wash and soak the mung dal and rice for a minimum of 30–60 minutes. Rinse and drain.
2. Heat the ghee in a medium saucepan. Add the cumin and whole spices, if using, and the turmeric and toast gently until aromatic (about 20 seconds).
3. Add the chopped onion and salt and allow to soften.
4. Add the pre-soaked rice and mung dal. Stir to coat the grains (1–2 minutes only).
5. Add the ginger, black pepper, bay leaf, chopped vegetables and hot water. Stir and bring to a boil. Reduce the heat, cover and simmer on medium heat for 30–45 minutes, stirring occasionally, until the grains and vegetables are softened. Add the chopped spinach after 30 minutes and let it wilt.
6. Adjust the consistency with additional hot water if needed – final consistency should resemble a thick porridge.
7. Add lemon juice and sprinkle with coriander then serve hot.

Ojas quinoa porridge

Quinoa is a light, complete-protein seed rich in magnesium and antioxidants, making it highly balancing for all *doṣas*. In this *rasāyana*-inspired porridge, quinoa builds strength, ghee supports digestion and tissue nourishment, and spices like cardamom and ginger gently kindle *agni*. Almonds, dates and saffron further enhance *ojas*, mood and cellular rejuvenation. You can also adapt this recipe with oats, rice or millet.

Serves 2

Ingredients:

- 100g (1 cup) quinoa
- 400ml (2 cups) water

→

- 250ml (1 cup) A2 organic cow's milk, almond milk or light coconut milk
- 1 tsp ghee (or tahini / coconut oil)
- ¼ tsp ground cinnamon
- ¼ tsp ground ginger
- pinch of ground cardamom (optional)
- 1 tbsp jaggery, to taste
- 1–2 soft dates, chopped, or 2 tbsp raisins (optional)
- pinch of saffron threads soaked in 1 tbsp warm milk (optional; highly *rasāyana*)
- flaked almonds, flaked coconut, pistachios, pumpkin or flax seeds, to garnish (optional)

Method:

1. Rinse the quinoa thoroughly under running water to remove any bitterness.
2. In a saucepan, combine the quinoa with the water. Bring to a boil, then reduce to medium–low heat and simmer for 15 minutes, stirring occasionally. Add the milk and continue to cook for 5–10 minutes.
3. Once the quinoa begins to soften, stir in the ghee, cinnamon, ginger, cardamom and jaggery. If you're adding dates, raisins or saffron milk, stir them in now.
4. Simmer gently until the porridge reaches a creamy, soft consistency. Add a splash of hot water if it thickens too much.
5. Turn off the heat and serve warm, topped with almonds and your choice of *rasāyana* garnishes.

Sattvic roasted butternut squash soup

This soft, velvety soup is made with sweet butternut squash and gentle *sattvic* spices. Designed to nourish digestion, calm the mind and build *ojas*, this is a simple recipe that supports deep tissue rejuvenation and emotional balance. Its natural sweetness and grounding qualities make it especially soothing during times of seasonal change or inner restoration. You can simplify the spicing using 1–2 tsp of a cumin,

→

coriander and fennel spice blend. I also love topping it with a handful of crispy oven-roasted kale.

Serves 3-4

Ingredients:

- 1 medium butternut squash, peeled, deseeded and cubed
- olive oil, salt and pepper (optional, for roasting)
- 1 tbsp ghee or coconut oil
- 1 tsp cumin seeds
- 1 onion, diced (optional)
- ½ tsp ground cinnamon
- 1 tsp grated fresh ginger
- ½ tsp fennel seeds (optional)
- ¼ tsp turmeric powder
- 750ml (3 cups) warm water or light vegetable broth
- 60ml (¼ cup) coconut milk (optional, for creaminess)
- 1 tsp mineral salt or rock salt (to taste)
- fresh coriander or parsley, finely chopped, to garnish

Method:

1. Preheat the oven to 180C fan° (200°C/gas 6). Roast the butternut squash with or without a little oil and a little salt and pepper for 35–40 minutes, or until the squash is tender and lightly golden.
2. Melt the ghee or coconut oil in a large heavy-bottomed pan over medium heat. Add the cumin seeds and let them sizzle for a few seconds. If using onions, add them now and cook for about 10 minutes, until softened.
3. Stir in the cinnamon, ginger, fennel seeds (if using) and turmeric. Let the spices bloom gently for about 20–30 seconds, without burning.
4. Add the roasted butternut squash and toss well to coat with the spiced ghee.
5. Pour in the warm water or broth. Bring to a gentle simmer.
6. Use a stick blender directly in the pan or transfer carefully to a blender and blend until smooth and creamy. Adjust the thickness by adding a little extra warm water if needed.
7. Stir in the coconut milk if using, then add salt to taste. Warm gently but do not boil after adding the coconut milk. Serve garnished with fresh coriander or parsley.

Pillar 3

Alchemy of youthfulness

> **'The doctor of the future will give no medicine but will interest his patients in the care of the human frame, diet, and in the cause and prevention of disease.'**
>
> **Thomas Edison**

It's quietly reassuring how nature always seems to provide exactly what we need, not only when we are sick, but also when we need deeper nourishment, strength and clarity. Herbs are nature's way of keeping us in balance and rooted in the earth. They help us stay connected to its cycles and keep our vitality on point. That's the promise of *rasāyana* herbs, tonics and formulas (*dravya rasāyana*).

In this pillar we focus on *dravya rasāyana*, the herbs, formulas and substances derived from nature's pharmacy. These include plants, roots, fruits, leaves, resins and mineral-rich substances that act as elixirs to restore vitality and longevity.

They don't just ease symptoms, they support proper tissue nourishment, starting with *rasa dhātu* (plasma), support *prāṇa* (life force), brighten *tejas* (inner radiance) and ultimately build *ojas*, the essence of immunity, resilience and vitality. Through a modern lens, many also act as natural antioxidants and anti-inflammatories, protecting the body from everyday wear and tear. Think of them as a mechanic who fixes the punctures in your tyres while ensuring your tank is also full for the journey ahead.

Rasāyana herbs are not designed to be quick fixes or anti-ageing hacks, but they serve as long-term herbal allies, helping us feel confident on the path of 'pro-ageing'.

Dravya rasāyanas become increasingly significant as we age. They play many roles, from keeping our joints supple and energy steady to enhancing memory, inner calm and even spiritual clarity.

In this pillar, we'll understand:

- How *dravya rasāyana* works and overlaps with the Western idea of adaptogens
- The key *rasāyana* herbs known for their pro-ageing properties, plus a quick-reference guide to some other beneficial herbs in the *rasāyana apothecary*
- Some of the key classical *rasāyana* formulas
- Some key considerations on sourcing herbs in a responsible, mindful way.

How *dravya rasāyanas* work

Dravya rasāyanas are not about popping a few herbs and hoping for the best. They are part of a larger alchemy of self-care that we are exploring through these seven pillars and work best when the foundations are stable - good digestion, clear channels and alignment with nature's rhythm. Herbs penetrate deeply only when *agni* is steady and the pathways of the body are flowing - remember, we can't truly nourish an already 'overloaded body'!

Dravya rasāyanas are not a one-size-fits-all solution or remedy for nutritional deficiency, they are preventative tonics that protect, strengthen and build long-term resilience. They work best when they are personalised to your unique constitution, what *Āyurveda* calls *yukti*. The *rasāyana* herbs you might need at the age of 30 in the winter could be very different to what your body craves at 50 in summer. They communicate with us at an energetic level and listening to the dialogue of the mind-body is part of their medicine.

To understand how *dravya rasāyanas* work, imagine a movie cast and crew:

- ***Dravya*** (the main actors) - herbal headliners like *amalaki* (Indian gooseberry) and *aśvagandhā* bring immunity, strength and vitality.
- ***Anupāna*** (the supporting roles) - carriers like ghee and milk help deliver herbs into the body, ensuring the main *dravya* shines.

- ***Yogavāhi*** (the directors behind the scenes) – substances like black pepper (*marica*) amplify and guide the action of the main *rasāyana* herb (*dravya*) to reach the deeper tissues.

Rasāyana herbs can be taken in many forms, but the most common is powders (*cūrṇa*), which is both accessible and considered superior to capsules or tablets. *Rasāyana* medicines also come as nourishing jams (*lehya*) – like *cyavanaprāśa*, medicated ghees (*ghṛtam*), decoctions (*kaṣāyam*) or simple teas and juices. Each *rasāyana* is paired with a delivery medium (*anupāna*) to help it absorb more effectively. The delivery medium is chosen to suit your constitution: warm water/milk or ghee is used to ground *vāta*; warm milk, ghee or cool water can be used to cool *pitta*; and honey, buttermilk or warm water to lighten *kapha*. Richer substances like ghee and jams are especially supportive in the cooler months when deep restoration is needed, while lighter teas, decoctions and juices are more digestible in the heat of summer.

Timing matters, too. *Rasāyana* herbs are most effective when digestion is clear and free of *āma,* and are best taken separately from meals. They are usually taken in the morning on an empty stomach, when *agni* is calm and receptive and food is not competing for transformation into the *dhātus*. Some nourishing *rasāyanas* are taken at bedtime, a natural time for tissue repair and *ojas* restoration. It's always best to consult a practitioner when it comes to taking herbs.

Many rasāyana herbs are anabolic in nature: they nourish, lubricate and are especially effective in calming *vāta*, the *doṣa* most prevalent as we age. Other *rasāyana* herbs rejuvenate by balancing and regulating – they enhance mind-body functions, reduce oxidative stress or support *prāna* and flow. Like all *rasāyana* practices, they require patience, and consistency goes a long way.

Bridging worlds: *rasāyana* and adaptogens

In today's fast-paced world, many *rasāyana* herbs are recognised under the modern label of adaptogens. Adaptogens help the body resist and adapt to stress at the physical, emotional and environmental levels, restoring balance rather than forcing change.

→

There's overlap between the two. Some *rasāyana*s are recognised as adaptogens, but not all adaptogens hold *rasāyana* status. Nevertheless, they both share the same sentiment of resilience and restoration.

Āyurveda's classic herbs, like *aśvagandhā*, *śatāvarī*, *amalaki* (Indian gooseberry) and *tulsi*, are celebrated as both a *rasāyana* and an adaptogen. Modern herbalism adds others you may recognise from teas and wellness blends: reishi (*Ganoderma lucidum*), chaga, cordyceps, maca, *Rhodiola rosea*, Siberian ginseng, schisandra - to name a few, along with nutrient dense plants such as cacao and moringa.

Although mushrooms were not traditionally used in *Āyurveda* and are sometimes considered *tamasic* (dulling), *Āyurveda* teaches us to judge a substance by its ***guṇa***, the true nature and quality of a substance. If something protects vitality and supports *ojas*, it can earn a place in modern *Āyurvedic* living.

Rasāyana apothecary

Now let's turn our attention to the *rasāyana* herbs themselves - the stars of the show, each with their own story, energetics and virtues that bolster the pro-ageing journey.

In this section, I'll walk you through a collection of some of my favourite timeless herbs known for their rejuvenating and *ojas* -promoting qualities. Each profile offers practical guidance on what the herb is used for, who it suits best and traditional ways to take it. With this knowledge, you can weave these magical treasures into your daily life - think of this as your *dravya rasāyana* reference guide, something to return to whenever you need inspiration. And if you want to go deeper, a practitioner can help you create more personalised blends that support your own unique path of pro-ageing. Note on herbal profiles: Each herb is introduced through its *Āyurvedic* energetic signature - *rasa* (taste), *guṇa* (qualities), ***vīrya*** (energetic potency), ***vipāka*** (post-digestive effect) and *doṣa* influence. This helps us to choose the most suitable herbs for the *prakṛti*, condition, age and season. These *rasāyanas* may be taken in the traditional powdered form (*cūrṇa*), usually ranging from 3-6g daily, introduced slowly (starting at a conservative 1.5g) and taken with an *anupāna* (such as water, milk, ghee or honey). These days, capsules and tablets are also available for convenience. The dosage and administration are individualised based on your constitution, goals and digestion, so they are not specified here. In *Āyurveda*, herbs are always used according to the context and function.

Amalaki (Indian gooseberry)

Botanical name: *Phyllanthus emblica*
Qualities (*guṇa*): Light (*laghu*), dry (*rūkṣa*)
Taste (*rasa*): All tastes except salty; predominantly sour
Potency (*vīrya*): Cooling (***śīta***)
Post-digestive effect (*vipāka*): Sweet (*madhura*)
Doṣa: ***Tridoṣa*** (balances all three *doṣas*)

Native to India, *amalaki* holds a sacred place in my *Āyurvedic* cabinet as a supreme *rasāyana*, a true gift for those who wish to age wisely and stay bright in mind and body. Its name means 'pure' or 'without stain', reflecting both its cleansing and life-giving nature. In the *Caraka Saṃhitā*, *amalaki* is called *'vayasthāpana'* (youth-preserving or revitalising) and *'jīvaniya'* (longevity-promoting). In the modern context it is emerging as a rejuvenative *rasāyana*, showing potential as a telomerase-modulating agent.

Rich in vitamin C (up to 10 times more than oranges), *amalaki* delivers antioxidants like emblicanin A & B, gallic acid and ascorbic acid, which combat free radicals, preserve cellular integrity and reduce oxidative stress. It is both nourishing and cleansing – a rare duality.

From an energetic standpoint, *amalaki* is cooling, grounding and stabilising, ideal for high *pittā* or frazzled *vāta*. Yet it balances all *doṣas* when used correctly, which is why it features in blends like *triphala* and *cyavanaprāśa*.

Amalaki is considered a pro-ageing powerhouse as it's great for:

- **Immunity**: Gently supports your body's natural defences, calms inflammation without overstimulation.

- **Vitality**: Rebuilds strength, supports adrenal health, enhances stamina.
- **Skin and hair**: Supports collagen, slows greying, restores glow.
- **Digestion**: Strengthens *agni*, cools acidity, improves absorption.
- **Cognition and heart**: Sharpens memory, may reduce LDL (low-density lipoprotein) cholesterol and trigycerides supporting vascular circulation.
- **Urinary and metabolic support**: Traditionally associated with healthy fluid metabolism, especially when combined with turmeric.

Traditional preparations:

- Fresh fruit or juice: Eat 1–2 fresh fruits daily or sip 10-30ml of juice for a rejuvenating kick (I recommend diluting with an equal amount of water). Fresh fruit offers greater bioavailability than powdered forms.
- *Amalaki* pulp can be prepared with ghee and honey and made into '*laddu*' energy balls or taken as a modern herbal jam (*Amlaprash*). *Āmalakī Rasāyana* is a classical rejuvenative preparation.
- Oil: Massage *amalaki*-infused oil into the scalp for strong, lustrous hair.

Aśvagandhā

Botanical name: *Withania somnifera*
Qualities (*guṇa*): Light (*laghu*), oily (*snigdha*)
Taste (*rasa*): Astringent (*kaṣāya*), bitter (***tikta***), sweet (*madhura*)
Potency (*vīrya*): Mildly heating (***uṣṇa***)
Post-digestive effect (*vipāka*): Sweet (*madhura*)
Doṣa: Pacifies *vāta* and *kapha*

Aśvagandhā, often called Indian ginseng or winter cherry, has surged in popularity in the West as a stress-relieving adaptogen, though its legacy in *Āyurveda* runs much deeper. *Aśvagandhā*, known in Sanskrit as 'smell of a horse', refers to its potent vitality-boosting power. It is said to give 'the strength of a stallion', both in physical vitality and in its ability to enhance virility; hence it is also labelled as a potent *vājīkaraṇa* (virility enhancer).

Traditionally used as a *bālya* (strengthener) for body and mind, *aśvagandhā* is one of the most powerful herbs for those navigating the changes and challenges of ageing, with emerging preclinical evidence suggesting it may influence stem-cell-related pathways and telomerase activity, alongside antioxidant and *rasāyana* effects. It tones the muscles, strengthens the reproductive system, calms the nerves and restores *ojas* resilience.

Aśvagandhā is the chosen adaptogen for modern life, great for:

- **Stress relief**: *Aśvagandhā* helps regulate cortisol and other stress hormones, easing the wear and tear caused by chronic stress and anxiety and supporting adrenal balance.
- **Energy and strength**: By supporting mitochondrial function and muscle tone, *aśvagandhā* restores stamina and energy. It's particularly effective for age-related debility, fatigue and sexual vitality, especially when taken with milk and ghee.
- **Cognition and mind**: *Aśvagandhā* enhances memory, focus and neuroplasticity. It is especially soothing for insomnia, stress-induced fatigue and tension.
- **Anti-inflammatory and antioxidant**: Rich in withanolides, *Aśvagandhā* helps reduce inflammation and oxidative stress – two key drivers of premature ageing and cellular decline.

Traditional preparations:

- Powder heated into warm milk (with a natural sweetener) as a tonic for balancing *vatā* and to promote sleep.
- Sauté the powder with ghee and jaggery to build strength, take with milk as an *anupāna*.
- Take as a tea infusion for a simple energy-balancing morning preparation.
- Can be consumed as a medicated ghee (*Aśvagandhā ghṛta*) for deeper tissue nourishment.
- *Aśvagandhā*-infused oil is perfect for massaging away *vāta*-related aches, debility and nervous exhaustion.

Bibhitaki

Botanical name: *Terminalia bellirica*
Qualities (*guṇa*): Light (*laghu*), dry (*rūkṣa*)
Taste (*rasa*): Astringent (*kaṣāya*)
Potency (*vīrya*): Heating (*uṣṇa*)
Post-digestive effect (*vipāka*): Sweet (*madhura*)
Doṣa: Balances *kapha* and *pittā*

Bibhitaki, the sharp and cleansing fruit of the *Terminalia bellirica* tree, forms one-third of the revered *triphala* formula, alongside *amalaki* and *haritaki*. While not a *rasāyana* in the classical sense, *bibhitaki* holds significant value in the *Āyurvedic* approach to pro-ageing. Its name refers to 'that which removes fear', hinting at its potent disease-fighting abilities.

This astringent fruit is an antioxidant powerhouse, packed with tannins and flavonoids that neutralise free radicals, slow down cellular degeneration and protect against chronic illness. Studies on *bibhitaki* point to its anti-inflammatory, antiviral and antimicrobial properties, important mechanisms in protecting health over time.

Bibhitaki is known as the cleanser and protector, great for:

- **Digestive and detox support**: *Bibhitaki* supports digestion and gentle gut cleansing: modern studies show it protects the intestinal lining and promotes regular bowel function, aligning with its traditional role of strengthening *agni* and clearing *āma* (toxins). Taken fresh (½ fruit), it relieves constipation, while powdered forms help calm loose motions, balancing elimination and digestive clarity.
- **Blood and skin purification**: By balancing *pittā* and supporting healthy blood, *bibhitaki* improves the complexion and calms skin flare-ups. It strengthens the hair and prevents premature greying.
- ***Ojas* and immunity building**: *Bibhitaki* purifies *kapha*-related stagnation, boosting immunity and resilience against respiratory infections and chronic imbalances.
- **Cognitive clarity**: In *Āyurveda, Bibhitaki's* astringent, light and drying qualities help reduce heaviness and sluggishness. *Bibhitaki* may also support memory and cognition, with

preclinical research in rats suggesting that its aqueous fruit extract may enhance learning and exert neuroprotective effects.
- **Lung and respiratory support**: Especially effective in clearing mucous and strengthening lung capacity, *bibhitaki* is useful in chronic cough, asthma and bronchial conditions.

Traditional preparation:

- Taken as a powder with warm water or with ghee to pacify *vatā* or as part of the *triphala* formula (*see also* p. 156).

Brahmi

Botanical name: *Bacopa monnieri*
Qualities (*guṇa*): Light (*laghu*), unctuous (*snigdha*)
Taste (*rasa*): Bitter (*tikta*), astringent (*kaṣāya*), sweet (*madhura*)
Potency (*vīrya*): Cooling (*śīta*)
Post-digestive effect (*vipāka*): Sweet (*madhura*)
Doṣa: Balances all three *doṣas*

It's only a matter of time until this best-kept *Āyurveda* secret reveals itself as the next wonder herb to the wider world. It's one that features regularly for me as I navigate perimenopause, when clarity, calm and emotional resilience are essential.

Brahmi, named after Saraswati, the goddess of wisdom, is *Āyurveda's* most beloved *medhya rasāyana* (brain and nervine tonic), elevating consciousness, emotional vitality and clinically proven useful for mental illness (*unmadahara*). It protects the nervous system from the effects of ageing and builds mental resilience. *Sattvic* in nature, it calms mental restlessness while sharpening the memory, learning, verbal expression and insight. It is as useful for reducing overthinking and anxiety as it is for enhancing focus and adaptability in later life (*medhya rasāyana*).

Brahmi is revered as the mind's rejuvenator, great for:

- **Neuroprotective and cognitive support**: *Brahmi* enhances neuroplasticity and synaptic communication. Studies show it boosts acetylcholine levels, improves memory retention and protects against age-related cognitive decline and neuroinflammation.

- **Emotional balance and stress relief**: *Brahmi* supports mood, restful sleep and emotional steadiness, so it's ideal for stress-prone *vāta* and *pittā* minds. Clinical and mechanistic studies show *brahmi*'s ability to lower the stress hormone cortisol and modulate serotonin, helping to reduce anxiety and elevate mood.
- **Cellular repair and longevity**: Research shows *brahmi* protects DNA from oxidative stress-induced damage, supporting cellular resilience and healthy ageing. *Brahmi* also reduces systemic inflammation and oxidative stress, key drivers in chronic conditions such as arthritis, diabetes and cardiovascular disease.
- **Skin and hair rejuvenation**: By enhancing collagen production and fibroblast activity, *brahmi* improves skin elasticity and supports cellular repair, helping to minimise fine lines and promote a healthy complexion. Traditionally, it is also applied as a scalp oil to soothe inflammation, strengthen hair follicles and slows premature greying.
- ***Ojas* and immune resilience**: *Sattvic* and cooling, *brahmi* supports *ojas* and balances the emotional body, making it a gentle yet potent ally for mind–body immunity. Modern research shows that *Brahmi* modulates cytokines and immune pathways, supporting its traditional role in building resilience.

Traditional preparations:

- Commonly prepared with milk or water or taken with honey or ghee in the morning for mental clarity.
- 10–20ml fresh juice diluted with a little warm water, honey or infused in warm milk.
- Available as a medicated ghee (*Brahmi ghṛta*) as a nervine tonic.
- Use *brahmi* oil for head and scalp massage to calm the mind, reduce stress and promote healthy hair.

Guḍūcī

Botanical name: *Tinospora cordifolia*
Qualities (*guṇa*): Light (*laghu*)
Taste (*rasa*): Bitter (*tikta*), astringent (*kaṣāya*), pungent (*kaṭu*)
Potency (*vīrya*): Heating (*uṣṇa*)
Post-digestive effect (*vipāka*): Sweet (*madhura*)
Doṣa: Balances all three *doṣas*

According to myth, *guḍūcī*, or *giloy*, was considered *amṛta*, the nectar derived from the churning of the ocean, and it was said that anyone who drank it would become 'immortal'. *Guḍūcī* is celebrated as one of *Āyurveda's* most potent *rasāyana* herbs, with its climbing vines and heart-shaped leaves symbolising renewal and vitality. I often call it '*God-uchi*' for its extraordinary breadth as an immune-strengthening, stress-resisting and deeply rejuvenating herb.

With its antioxidant, adaptogenic and immunomodulatory properties, *guḍūcī* helps protect the body against oxidative stress and inflammation while supporting cellular health. In *Āyurveda*, it promotes *ojas* and longevity. As part of a holistic approach, this plant is used to support immunity and to help maintain resilience against age-related disorders such as diabetes and arthritis, while also supporting bone and muscle health.

Guḍūcī is celebrated as the nectar of immortality, great for:

- **Immunity and resilience**: *Guḍūcī* modulates immune function, reducing chronic inflammation while increasing resistance to viral infections. Clinical and preclinical studies indicate its efficacy in supporting recovery from fevers like dengue, influenza and even Covid-19.
- **Detoxification and rejuvenation**: It purifies the blood, clears *āma* (toxins) and supports *dhātu* integrity and vitality from within. Its bitter and light qualities make it particularly supportive for *kapha*-related sluggishness, poor digestion and lymphatic congestion.
- **Joint and bone support**: When processed with ghee or milk, *guḍūcī* is traditionally used to support the bones and joints and ease age-related stiffness.

- **Cognitive clarity**: As a *medhya rasāyana*, *guḍūcī* supports mental clarity, memory and perception, while shielding the brain from oxidative stress and cognitive decline.
- **Skin and hair health**: Its antioxidant properties help supports healthy skin ageing and improves dull-looking skin.

Traditional preparations:

- A starch extract made from the plant stems (*Guḍūcī satva*) - taken with milk or honey.
- Make a decoction by boiling dried stem powder in water or take powder with warm water, milk or honey.
- Taken as a medicated ghee (*Guḍūcī ghṛta*) - indicated in chronic inflammation.
- Drink 10-20ml fresh juice extracted by crushing and soaking stems.

Haritaki

Botanical name: *Terminalia chebula*
Qualities (*guṇa*): Light (*laghu*), dry (*rūkṣa*)
Taste (*rasa*): All five tastes except salty; predominantly astringent (*kaṣāya*)
Potency (*vīrya*): Heating (*uṣṇa*)
Post-digestive effect (*vipāka*): Sweet (*madhura*)
Doṣa: Balances all three; may aggravate *pittā* in excess

Haritaki, the 'king of herbs', essentially means 'the one who takes away diseases' - a potent *and* poetic name for a fruit so integral in *dravya rasāyana*. Perhaps we can associate '*Hara*' with Lord Shiva, suggesting this plant carries the energy of dissolution and renewal. Sometimes called the 'Indian walnut', it is one of the three musketeers of *triphala* and central to digestive and systemic rejuvenation.

With its wrinkled green rind resembling the brain, *haritaki* has been praised for enhancing wisdom, longevity and sharpness of perception. Its astringent taste and light, dry nature give it powerful detoxifying abilities, especially through the gut and colon. It rejuvenates and balances the body's three *doṣas* (only aggravating *pittā* if taken in excess).

Haritaki is honoured as the great cleanser, especially good for:

- **Digestive and detox support**: *Haritaki* gently regulates elimination, acting as both a mild laxative and a digestive tonic depending on the dose. Research shows it supports gut motility and helps protect the intestinal mucosa, mirroring its traditional role in clearing *āma* (toxins) and supporting *agni* (digestive fire).
- **Antioxidant protection**: Rich in tannins and vitamin C, *haritaki* protects cells from oxidative stress and inflammation, two key drivers of ageing and chronic disease, by modulating antioxidant pathways and inflammatory mediators.
- **Immune strength**: Its antimicrobial and anti-inflammatory properties can support immune resilience and help reduce susceptibility to chronic conditions.
- **Cognitive and sensory clarity**: As a *medhya rasāyana*, *haritaki* sharpens memory and intellect while nourishing the sensory organs, especially vision, speech and hearing – yes, please! Research shows it protects brain tissue from oxidative damage and may help delay age-related cognitive decline.
- **Metabolic Balance**: *Harītakī* is traditionally used to help clear excess *kapha* and *meda*, supporting metabolic balance in conditions such as obesity and diabetes.

Traditional preparations:

- Taken as a powder with warm water or milk for digestive and immune support, add ghee for *vatā* balancing.
- Prepared as a *Murabba* – a herbal jam made with fresh *haritaki* fruit cooked with spices in a jaggery syrup.

Śatāvarī

Botanical name: *Asparagus racemosus*
Qualities (*guṇa*): Heavy (*guru*), oily (*snigdha*)
Taste (*rasa*): Bitter (*tikta*), sweet (*madhura*)
Potency (*vīrya*): Cooling (*śīta*)
Post-digestive effect (*vipāka*): Sweet (*madhura*)
Doṣa: Pacifies *vāta* and *pittā*

A gorgeous, well-loved root herb, *śatāvarī* is called the 'Queen of herbs' and is one of *Āyurveda's* most revered *rasāyanas* for women. And rightly so, since it has long been used to support hormonal balance and vitality through life's major transitions, from menstruation and conception to pregnancy, perimenopause and menopause. This must be why *śatāvarī* means 'the plant with 100 roots' or 'she who has 100 husbands'.

Found throughout India, this gentle root is part of the asparagus family and as a *sattvic*, adaptogenic herb, *śatāvarī* supports the body by adapting to emotional and hormonal stress.

I recommend *śatāvarī* for many clients facing everything from amenorrhoea and PMS to infertility, hot flushes and postpartum depletion. Its rich, unctuous and cooling nature deeply nourishes the reproductive system, builds *ojas* and supports mental calm.

Śatāvarī is cherished as the great nourisher of feminine energy, especially beneficial for:

- **Hormonal harmony**: *Śatāvarī* supports healthy oestrogen and progesterone balance, easing PMS, perimenopausal and menopausal symptoms like hot flushes, dryness and mood fluctuations. Traditionally, it is also used to enhance vitality and libido in menopausal women.
- **Adaptogenic resilience:** *Śatāvarī* helps the body adapt to stress, eases fatigue and supports immune balance through its proven anti-stress and restorative actions.
- **Digestive and metabolic support**: Soothes ulcers and inflammation, regulates healthy digestion and has been shown in studies to help regulate blood sugar and cholesterol levels.
- **Skin and vitality**: As a *rasāyana, shatavari* supports healthy ageing by nourishing the tissues and promoting strength and endurance.
- **Nervous system and emotional nourishment**: Soothes the nerves, calms anxiety and strengthens emotional resilience, especially during hormonal transitions. Recent research confirms its adaptogenic and neuroprotective actions, helping the body and mind adapt to stress. *Śatāvarī* is considered *hṛdaya* – nourishing the emotional heart and supporting creative impulses.

Traditional preparations:

- Take powder boiled in milk taken warm for general vitality and female hormone regulation (honey or jaggery can be used to sweeten) - *see* Śatāvarī-rose *soma* milk recipe, pp. 134–5.
- A medicinal ghee (*Śatāvarī grita*) is a great for women's health and overall vitality.
- Made into a jam preparation with jaggery (*Śatāvarī gulam*) and taken with warm milk.

Additional notable *dravya rasāyanas*

In addition to the well-known *rasāyana* herbs we've just explored, there are many others that support resilience, longevity and inner nourishment. To keep things practical, I've gathered them in Table 8.1 below - a quick-reference guide you can dip into whenever you want to discover new *rasāyana* allies (including some Western options).

Herb	Key benefit
Kumari (aloe vera)	Soothes digestion and cools inflammation, great for skin. Moistens and opens channels; supports absorption, especially women's health. Also a *yogavahi*.
Bala (country mallow)	Strengthens nerves and boosts vitality.
Bṛṅgarāja (false daisy)	Revitalises hair and nourishes the liver.
Gotu kola (Indian pennywort)	Boosts memory and calms the mind.
Guggulu (Indian Myrrh)	Cleanses tissues and supports joints. Channel-opener and detoxifier; carries herbs to joints and tissues.
Pippalī (long pepper)	Enhances bioavailability and clears lungs.
Hawthorn (May tree)	Strengthens the heart (cardiotonic) and improves circulation (Western adaptogen).

Herb	Key benefit
Laśuna (garlic)	Lowers cholesterol and clears channels.
Śaṅkhapuṣpī (morning glory)	Nourishes the brain and eases anxiety.
Śilājit (mineral exudate)	Restores energy, boosts immunity and supports cognitive function. Deep-penetrating catalyst; enhances absorption of mineral and herbal *rasāyana*.
Rhodiola rosea (arctic root)	Boosts energy, builds stress resilience and has anti-cancer properties (Western adaptogen).
Punarnavā (spreading hogweed)	Acts as a natural diuretic to reduce water retention and supports kidney rejuvenation.
Haridrā (turmeric)	A protective antioxidant spice that fights inflammation and supports immunity.
Tulasī (holy basil)	Protects lungs and strengthens immunity.
Yaṣṭimadhu (liquorice)	Soothes mucosa and supports adrenal health.

Table 8.1 Notable *dravya rasāyanas*

If *rasāyana* herbs are the stars of the show, the directors (*yogavāhīs*) intelligently help the actors (*rasāyana* herbs) to work more deeply without losing their own virtue. They guide nourishment to the right places (*dhātus*), amplify potency, enhancing absorption and bringing harmony to the whole formula. A few common *yogavāhī* ingredients include: *Śuṇṭhī* (dry ginger), *Marica* (black pepper), *Pippalī* (long pepper), *Trikatu* (a blend of the previous three), *Madhu* (honey) and *Saindhava* (rock salt).

Classical *rasāyana* formulas

There are many potent *rasāyana* formulas containing ingredients such as *bhasmas* – purified metal or mineral preparations that are traditionally used in *Āyurvedic* alchemy (*rasāśāstra*) but not so common (or suitable for everyone) today. In practice today, there are several well-known and easily available *rasāyana* blends, including *triphala*, *brahma rasāyana*, *cyavanaprāśa* and *amṛta kalaśa to name a few*. Here are two of my most versatile favourites (*see* Resources, pp. 271–2, for herbal suppliers):

Triphala

My favourite showstopper, this is the first formula I learned about and one that continues to hold the number one spot in my herbal charts. I just can't get enough of it, and neither will you once you unveil its benefits. It combines the collective intelligence of *amalaki*, *haritaki* and *bibhitaki*, as we saw in the previous pages, bringing a full spectrum of support for long-term vitality.

More than just the digestive tonic it is known for, *triphala* is a 360° *rasāyana*, a rejuvenator for the tissues, the gut, the mind and the spirit. It strengthens the process of cellular repair, protects against oxidative stress and enhances *ojas* and immune resilience.

As a pro-ageing ally, *triphala* works behind the scenes but powerfully to slow degeneration, nourish the deeper layers of the body and maintain internal balance. Taken regularly, it helps the body self-correct before imbalance manifests into disease, making it an essential choice for pro-ageing.

It's rich in antioxidants and has anti-inflammatory, antibacterial and antiviral properties, making it a true guardian of longevity. For anyone looking to enhance digestion, metabolism, immunity or to simply feel lighter and brighter, *triphala* is a daily tonic worth embracing. Since it can be slightly drying, especially for *vāta* types, it is sometimes combined with ghee and warm water for balance. This formula is widely available through health food stores and online *Āyurvedic* suppliers (*see* Resources, pp. 271–2, for details).

How to incorporate: Traditionally, this *tridoshic* blend would be taken with ghee and/or honey and followed with warm water or as a powder in warm water before bed or first thing in the morning. *Triphala* can also be used externally as a hair and skin tonic.

Cyavanaprāśa – a vitality tonic

If there's one *dravya rasāyana* formula that feels like a big bear hug for the whole body, it's *cyavanaprāśa*. This luscious dark herbal jam has been treasured for thousands of years as a *rasāyana* elixir, designed to nourish, strengthen and bring lasting vitality through every stage of life.

At its heart is *amalaki*, one of the richest natural sources of vitamin C, blended with around 50 ingredients: herbs, spices, ghee, honey and sesame oil to create a 'lickable medicine' that's both delicious and deeply restorative. *Cyavanaprāśa* is rich in antioxidants, supports immunity, vitality and resistance to infections. It enhances digestion, assimilation and metabolism while building strength, stamina and muscle tone - making it an ideal tonic for colder months when the energy of *vāta* can leave us feeling dry, tired or depleted.

Rather than simply replacing what's missing, *cyavanaprāśa* works by supporting the body's natural intelligence. It rekindles *agni* (digestive fire), clears *āma* (toxins) and nourishes *ojas* (vitality and immunity) - bolstering all those things we are working on through the other six pillars. Minus the salty taste, it's a perfect blend of sweet, sour, bitter, astringent and pungent that delights the palate, while deeply grounding your whole system.

How to incorporate: Enjoy one teaspoon daily straight from the jar (a great swap for Nutella), or with warm water as a shot (how I have mine), or even spread on toast. Then let this ancient formula weave its magic through your body and mind (*see* Resources, pp. 271–2, for suppliers).

Āyurvedic anti-inflammatory support

So, we know that chronic inflammation is one of the key culprits that hasten ageing and it is usually caused by an impaired *agni* (metabolic fire), which gives rise to *āma* (toxins) as well as *doṣa* imbalances. It can show up as heaviness, aches or pains in the body: maybe your joints feel stiff in the morning, or your digestion just isn't as clear and light as it used to be. You might notice your skin acting up, your energy feeling a bit foggy, or an emotional irritability that's hard to shake off. If this feels like you, before you focus on anabolic *rasāyana* foods and herbs, it may serve you to initially focus on reducing the inflammatory build-up and take on a gentle cleanse (*see* 'Stimulating the digestive fire' in chapter 5, p. 77). To bolster this process, you can opt to include *triphala* and *trikatu* (a pungent digestive herbal formula) or create your own anti-inflammatory formula with ingredients such as *āmalakī*, *haridrā* (turmeric), *śuṇṭhī* (dry ginger), *marica* (black pepper), coriander, *yaṣṭimadhu* (liquorice), *guḍūcī, mañjiṣṭhā, eranda* (castor) etc. Many are to be found in your home store cupboard.

Rasāyana herbs usage tips

- Gentle *rasāyanas - amla, brahmi, guḍūcī, aśvagandhā, śatāvarī, triphala* and *cyavanaprāśa* - are safe for regular use in small doses over longer periods provided *agni* is stable.
- Some herbs are more intense than others and are best taken used cyclically, for weeks at a time, under practitioner guidance.
- It is best to take your *rasāyana* herbs with a suitable carrier in the morning on an empty stomach and only eat breakfast once it has digested.
- *Panchakarma,* or a gentle system cleanse and reset can support absorption - *see* 'Stimulating the digestive fire' in chapter 5, p. 77.
- Follow *dinacaryā*, time-restricted eating and portion control to maximise efficacy - see chapter 5 and pillar 1.
- Always consult a qualified *Āyurvedic* practitioner or herbalist for dosage and duration instructions, based on your individual needs, especially if you're using more potent *rasāyana*s.

Cautions and contraindications

Avoid taking *rasāyana* herbs and formulas:

- Right after a heavy meal (you can have them at the start)
- During periods of acute illness or stress
- Without first addressing poor digestion or toxin build-up (*āma*)
- If you have high kapha (heaviness, loss of appetite, coated tongue, indigestion, irritability, sluggish bowels) or *kapha*-related conditions
- If you're pregnant, lactating, on medication or managing chronic conditions, consult an *Āyurvedic* practitioner.

Sourcing with awareness

As the popularity of *Āyurvedic* herbs grows around the world, so too does the pressure on Mother Nature's supply chain. Many *rasāyana* plants like *aśvagandhā* and *śatāvarī* are now well sought after, raising concerns around overharvesting, habitat loss and unsustainable farming practices.

Sadly, these sacred plants, traditionally gathered with care and respect for nature, are increasingly subject to mass cultivation and sometimes without regard for soil health, biodiversity or regeneration. So do take this into consideration when choosing herbs and take time to research whether there are local herbs with similar properties that may be available near you. For example, echinacea and astragalus can support immunity like *guḍūcī*, *Dong Quai* can nourish the female system like *śatāvarī*, *Rhodiola* can build resilience like *aśvagandhā* and elderberry can potentially protect and rejuvenate like *amalaki*.

When choosing brands and comparing price points of herbs, it's worth verifying: *what part of the plant is used?* For example, *aśvagandhā* root is considered the most potent part, but some cheaper products use leaves or stems instead, altering both quality and efficacy.

Understanding what you're consuming and where it came from creates a more intimate connection with the herbs and honours the wisdom they carry. When our healing choices align with nature, we not only support our own longevity, but also the longevity of the plants, ecosystems and cultural heritage, allowing future generations to benefit for years to come.

Pillar 4

Resilience and radiance rituals

'The yogi conquers the body by the practice of asanas and makes it a fit vehicle for the spirit.'

B.K.S. Iyengar

We've been taught to measure beauty by how well we preserve our youthful looks, comparing ourselves to who we were 10, 20, 30 years ago, or to someone else our age who seems to have 'aged-less' or 'aged better'. Physical ageing is a natural process we should embrace rather than resist or compare. That said, caring for our outer shell in a mindful, natural way isn't vanity, it's an act of honouring the body that we live in. A true beauty regimen begins with rituals from the inside and out, no matter which season of life you are in. So, through pillar 4, we will explore rituals to take good care of your body at a physical level, including:

- Mindful movement and benefits of functional fitness to sustain a strong mind and the body
- My 10 favourite pro-ageing yoga poses
- Natural skincare from the inside and out for the face and body
- Holistic haircare
- How to navigate the increasingly toxic environments we live in.

Conscious movement mastery

Vyayāma, meaning mindful exercise and conscious movement, builds strength and stamina when practised in moderation. It feels most powerful when it's aligned with your unique constitution (*prakruti*), the season and your body's capacity. In the context of longevity, gentle, regular movement truly is medicine. Our modern lives are more sedentary than ever, and I say this with awareness, especially as I find myself sitting for long stretches while writing these very reflections. Numerous studies have shown that prolonged sedentary time is linked to increased risk of cardiovascular disease, Type 2 diabetes, cancer, obesity, metabolic syndrome, musculoskeletal disorders and all-cause mortality, even after accounting for physical activity levels.

As we age, *vāta* (air and space qualities) naturally increases, bringing with it a greater tendency towards stiffness, reduced muscle tone and joint sensitivity. This makes regular movement more essential, not less. The right kind of exercise helps maintain strength, flexibility and vitality, gently protecting against frailty. *Yoga* ***āsanas*** are a conscious form of movement that nurtures balance, circulation and resilience, while staying deeply connected to breath and awareness. When combined with intention, *prāṇāyāma* (breathwork and energy regulation) and meditation, it becomes a powerful way to ease stress and encourage harmony of body, mind and spirit.

From an *Āyurvedic* perspective, exercise is about more than just physical mobility and muscles: it is to enhance *ojas* (vital essence), balance *agni* (metabolic fire) and support the *srotas* (body channels) by maintaining proper circulation and prevent the accumulation of *āma* (toxins). It also promotes mental clarity and emotional stability. Exercise supports holistic health by improving mood, lowering cortisol levels and enhancing neuroplasticity, and contributes to mental health and longevity.

Bearing this in mind, here are some *Āyurvedic* tips to help you move in a way that supports graceful ageing, nourishes *ojas* and honours your unique constitution:

- **Exercise to half your capacity** (*ardha śakti*). You should feel energised, not exhausted – overexertion can cause depletion of *ojas*. Signs of pushing too hard include fatigue, dryness and breathlessness. Wearable fitness trackers while exercising can help you stay well within your maximum heart rate limit.
- **Exercise in the morning.** 6 to 10 a.m. is ideal, when *kapha* energy is highest. This is when cortisol levels are naturally higher and the body is more stable, energetic and ready for activity.

- **Match intensity to the season.** In summer, opt for gentle walks, swimming or cooling yoga. In winter, try more dynamic movements like strength training or cardio.
- **Focus on the breath** during movement, as this improves oxygenation, energy flow and mental calm, hence why breath leads yoga *āsana* practice.
- **Avoid exercising right after eating** - though a gentle walk is fine. Give yourself two to three hours after a main meal before exercising to avoid disrupting digestion, otherwise it could lead to bloating, acid reflux or toxin (*āma*) formation. Exercise is best done when digestion feels clear and the body feels light. For some, that's an empty stomach, for others, a light snack such as a piece of fresh fruit or a date with soaked almonds in the morning can give a little energy support. Or how about a teaspoon of *cyavanaprāśa*? (*See* pillar 3).
- **Wait at least 20–30 minutes after exercise to eat.** This allows your energy to settle and ground again after intense activity and before digestion begins. Choose warm, easy-to-digest and protein/fat-rich foods such as rice, lentils, vegetables, nuts, seeds and ghee to replenish the tissues and restore energy. Avoid chilled drinks and cold foods at this time. A warm milk tonic with ghee and herbs, such as *aśvagandhā* and/or *śatāvarī*, helps the body repair after exertion.
- **Avoid heavy evening meals after workouts**, otherwise they strain digestion and divert energy away from muscle repair and hormone balance (cortisol, adrenaline and insulin), making recovery less effective.
- **Embrace energetic movement** like dancing, flowing yoga and hip-opening exercises to support the *nādīs* (subtle energy channels), and *chakras* like the sacral centre (*svādhisthāna*), encouraging creativity and sensuality.
- **Engage in group activities** such as walking clubs, dance, team or racquet sports or yoga sessions. Moving together encourages community connection and playfulness - nurturing emotional well-being and reducing stress.

Size and weight factor

We may look the same size as we did years ago, but what's happening beneath the surface often tells a different story. As we age, muscle mass naturally declines, even if our weight stays the same or drops. Often, it's muscle, not fat that we're losing, which can affect our strength, energy and resilience over time. So be mindful of what the scales are telling you; they only offer a limited picture.

An incidental exercise mindset

Do we really need expensive gym memberships? Adopting more incidental and dynamic movement can be the best form of exercise – it just becomes part of your every day and this can include sitting on the floor for meals or meditation, taking the stairs instead of the lift and a gentle walk after meals. It can also include gardening, dancing, house chores, playing with kids or walking barefoot on the grass or earth. If you are desk-bound, periodic movement, such as standing, stretching, squatting while you wait for the kettle to boil or taking short walks also helps maintain vitality – or have you tried using a standing desk? Studies on NEAT (Non-Exercise Activity Thermogenesis) highlight that incidental movement throughout the day contributes significantly to calorie expenditure and metabolic health. This is after all how our ancestors would have 'worked out'!

Exercise as medicine

In our modern-day sedentary living, incidental movement may not feel enough, so we need to consider more purposeful exercise that is joyful, functional and medicinal for pro-ageing while respecting our age and energy levels. Let's dive deeper into some things to consider when deciding what exercise is right for you.

Have you ever been in a fitness class and felt like you couldn't keep up? You're not alone. Exercise should be personal and aligned with your body type, age, environment and the season. Not everyone is built to run marathons, and that's OK. What matters more is finding a rhythm that works for you. Exercise should leave you feeling energised, lightly hungry, clear and mentally alert, supporting *ojas* formation. It should not leave you feeling thirsty, depleted, exhausted, or irritable.

Too much of a good thing can also imbalance us! Sometimes moderation, balance and consistency are more powerful than intensity. Even light activity can extend lifespan, as shown in a study from the *American Journal of Preventive Medicine*, which found that small increases in daily movement significantly improved longevity, especially for less active individuals.

The key is choosing movement that you truly enjoy and can sustain. Whether it's yoga, walking, dancing, strength training or swimming, let it be something that brings you joy. That's when movement becomes medicine and for me, that's brisk walking in the woods.

Pro-ageing tip: 'green exercise'

Try doing physical activity in the calming environment of nature. It can be anything that you choose but being outdoors soothes the nervous system and balances *vāta*.

As we age, loss of muscle mass is inevitable and this could be our greatest risk factor. Leg muscles and core strength may just be the two most important factors for maintaining mobility and longevity, since these are the muscle groups that we are going to need into our ripe old age. You don't need an hour, a gym or fancy equipment, just 10 to 15 minutes, your body and some floor space. It's not about aesthetics or burning calories. It's about staying functional and independent, for getting out of bed without help, standing up from a chair with ease, squatting comfortably to use the loo and lifting your grandchild (or your shopping) without a grimace.

My daily go-to pro-ageing exercise routine

I worked with a personal trainer (PT) who helped me start doing low-impact resistance training, weights and dynamic movement that mimicked the way different animals move – it was mind-blowingly impactful.

A qualified personal trainer can be invaluable to get you started and/or stay on track. Whether you are a fan of the gym or prefer low-key home workouts, here's what I recommend, including (but not exclusively) in your exercise plan whatever your age:

Exercise	Key benefits
Squats	Strengthen legs, glutes and the core. Help maintain mobility in the hips and knees – essential for sitting and standing with ease.
Lunges	Improve balance, co-ordination and leg strength. Keeps gait stable and joints aligned.
Deadlifts (with light weights or even water bottles)	Strengthen the back, glutes and hamstrings. Great for preventing back injuries and improving posture.
Plank	Builds core stability, supports the spine and enhances overall strength. Since this is a static pose, try holding for 30 seconds and build up to one minute.
Crunches or slow bicycle twists	Strengthen abdominal muscles, improve digestion and support lower back health.
Wall push-ups or incline push-ups	Strengthen the upper body, maintain shoulder mobility and keep the chest open.
Superman holds	Strengthen the lower back and glutes and improve spinal alignment. Hold this static pose for 30–60 seconds.
Toe raises and ankle circles	Improve circulation and joint mobility and help prevent falls.
Marching (optional: high knee marching)	Improves balance and gait, gently raises heart rate, strengthens legs and hips. Increase/decrease intensity to suit.

Table 9.1 Exercises and their benefits

Yoga for ageless living

'You are as young as your spine is flexible,' said Joseph Pilates, reflecting the sentiment of how yoga supports long-term physical health and more. Yoga has been proven to reduce markers of inflammation, improve flexibility and support mental well-being, making it an ideal movement practice for pro-ageing. All yoga *āsanas* bring huge health benefits but here are my top 10 yoga postures for pro-ageing. I've chosen these postures to support every system of the body – muscles, hormones, digestion, circulation and the mind, creating a steady foundation for longevity and *Rasāyana* living.

> **'Yoga is the journey of the self, through the self, to the self.'**
> ***Popular paraphrase inspired by the Bhagavad Gītā 6.20-23***

Ten pro-ageing yoga *āsanas*

1. ***Padmāsana* (Lotus Pose)**
   A meditative posture with crossed legs and the feet resting on the opposite thighs.

   Benefits: Promotes mental clarity, calms the nervous system and balances *prāṇa* flow – essential for sustaining vitality.

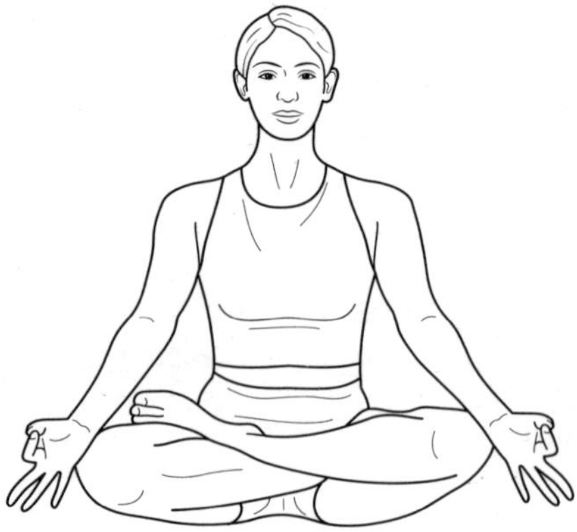

2. ***Siddhāsana* (Perfect Pose)**

A seated posture with one heel pressing the perineum and the other foot placed in front.

Benefits: Opens the subtle energy channels (*nādīs*), supports diaphragmatic breathing and deepens focus, enhancing longevity through stillness.

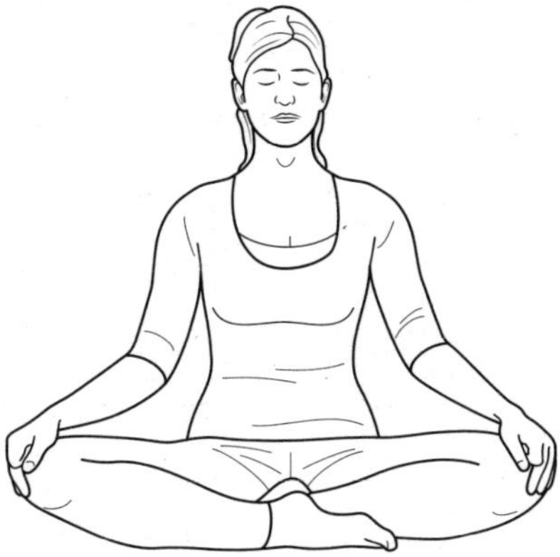

3. ***Tāḍāsana* (Mountain Pose)**

A standing posture that engages the whole body, grounding through the feet while lengthening the spine.

Benefits: Encourages postural alignment, balance and circulation; strengthens the legs and spine, encouraging confidence and stability.

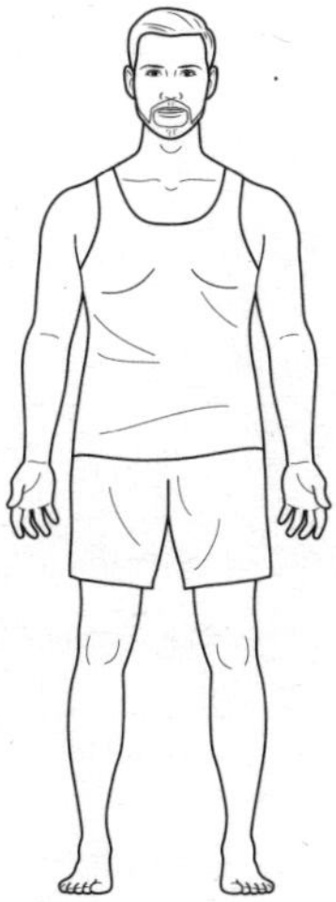

4. ***Matsyāsana* (Fish Pose)**
A gentle heart- and throat-opening backbend, reclining with the chest lifted and the crown resting lightly on the mat.

Benefits: Stimulates the thyroid and pituitary function, opens the chest and lungs, and enhances oxygenation – promoting hormonal harmony and resilience.

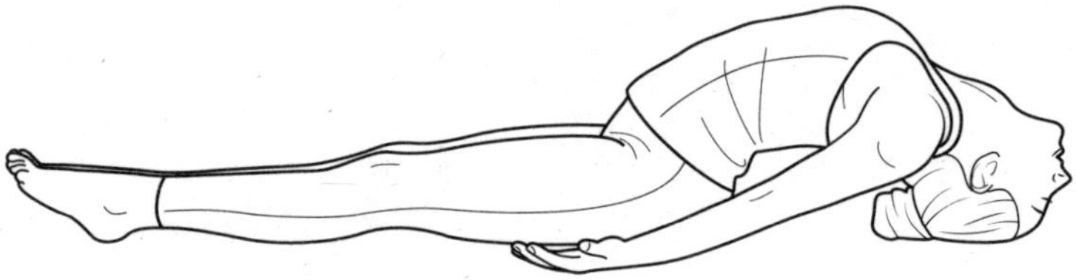

5. ***Marjaryāsana/Bitilāsana* (Cat/Cow Pose)**
A flowing sequence alternating between spinal flexion *Marjaryāsana* (Cat Pose), and spinal extension *Bitilāsana* (Cow Pose), as the spine rounds and gently dips.

Benefits: Promotes spinal flexibility, improves circulation and soothes the nervous system to alleviate ageing-related stiffness.

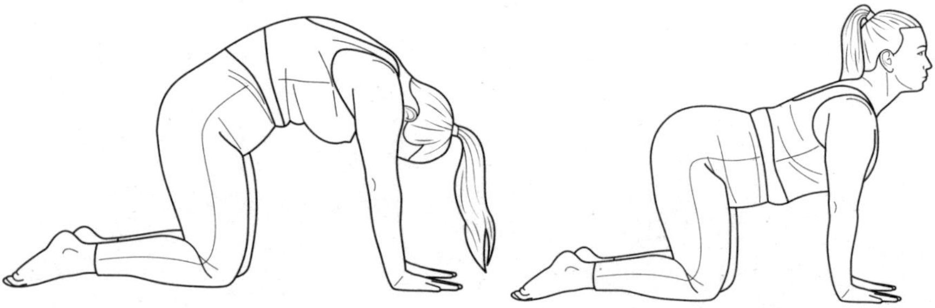

6. ***Paścimottānāsana* (Seated Forward Bend)**
   A seated forward bend over extended legs.

   Benefits: Stimulates digestion and detoxification, stretches the spine and calms the mind for deep restoration.

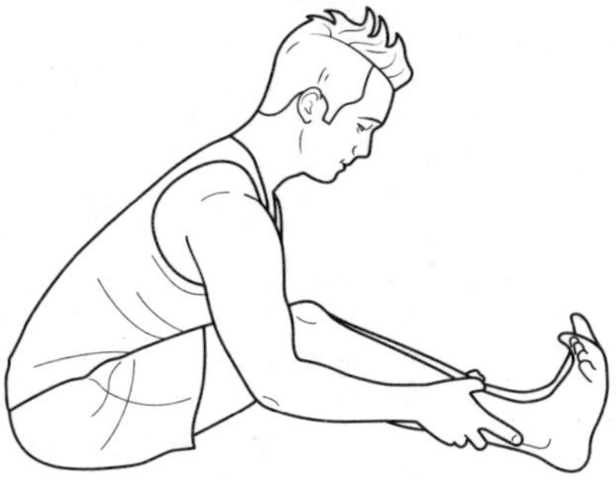

7. ***Ardha Matsyendrāsana* (Half Spinal Twist)**
   A seated twist where one leg is bent and the opposite arm crosses the knee, twisting the torso back over the shoulder.

   Benefits: Supports digestion, tones abdominal organs and enhances spinal mobility, promoting detoxification and rejuvenation.

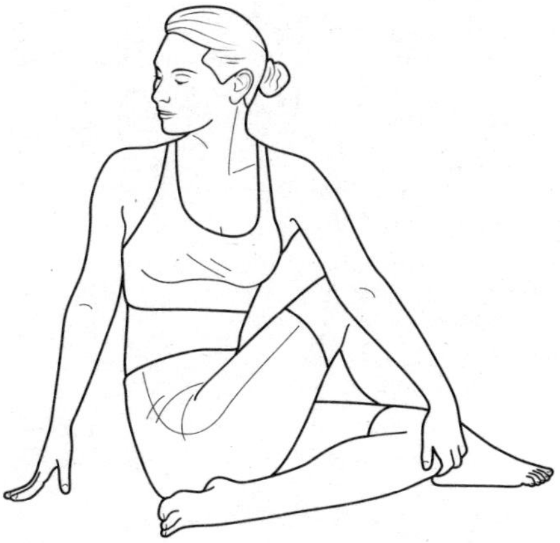

8. ***Bhujaṅgāsana* (Cobra Pose)**
A prone backbend lifting the chest and head while keeping the pelvis grounded.

Benefits: Strengthens the spine, balances stress hormones and improves digestion and circulation for tissue regeneration.

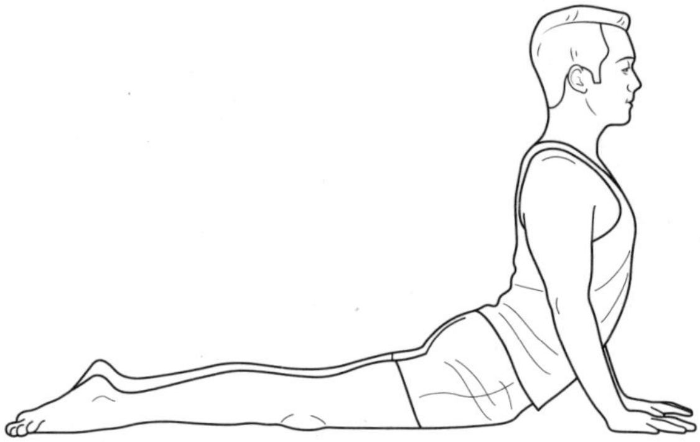

9. ***Viparīta Karaṇī* (Legs Up the Wall Pose)**
A restorative inversion with legs extended vertically up a wall while the back rests on the floor.

Benefits: Enhances circulation, reduces swelling and inflammation, calms the nervous system and restores *ojas* (vitality).

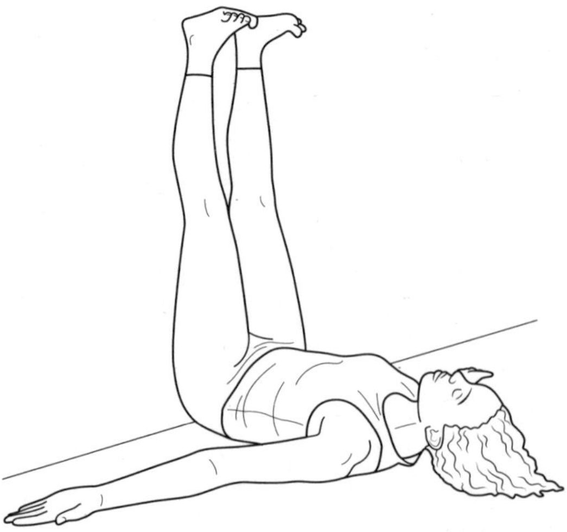

10. ***Śavāsana* (Corpse Pose)**

The long-awaited pose at the end of a class. A fully reclined posture that supports deep rest and awareness.

Benefits: Facilitates deep relaxation, activates the body's healing response and integrates the benefits of other poses for overall health.

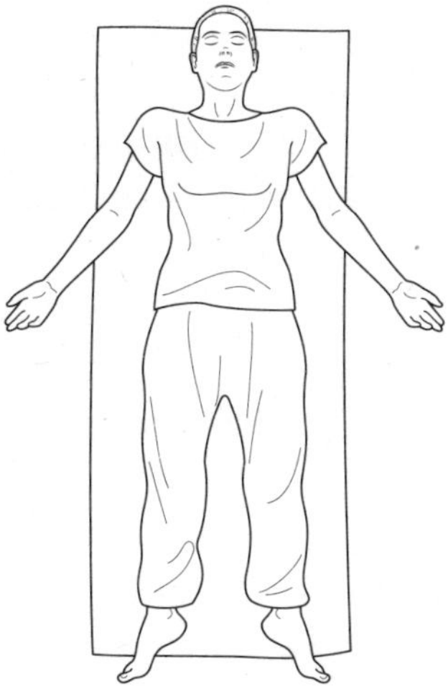

Pro-ageing exercise: practise sitting on the floor every day

There are many seated yoga *āsanas* – *Padmāsana*, *Siddhāsana*, *Vajrāsana* and *Sukhāsana*. You can choose whichever one feels natural but try to sit on the floor every day. Whether you're eating, reading or watching TV, this simple practice helps improve posture, supports digestion and keeps the hips, knees and lower back flexible, which is especially important as we age.

I remember family gatherings where we'd sit cross-legged on the floor regardless of age, eating with our hands and without distraction. It wasn't just about food: it was grounding, humbling and communal. Getting up and down from the floor regularly has even been linked to greater mobility and longevity. It's a small act, but over time, it keeps the body supple and our spirit grounded.

The importance of rest periods

After periods of exercise, rest and rejuvenation is an essential part of the conscious movement mix. This is why *Śavāsana* is integrated into almost all yoga classes and *abhyanga* (warm oil massage) is encouraged in *Āyurveda*. Recovery periods post-exercise allow for muscle repair, hormonal and energy regulation and encourage mental resilience. Overtraining without adequate rest can be counterproductive in the process of pro-ageing.

Do what you can and do it daily. Even a round of the workout routine or *asāna* practices I have included here can help you build muscle mass, support bone density and keep *agni* (metabolic fire) active.

Body beautiful

Your gut, liver, intestines and colon are constantly working to digest food, absorb nutrients and eliminate what your body doesn't need. This supports the body's natural detoxification, keeping your system flowing and your energy clear.

Your skin, often overlooked, plays a vital role too. As your largest organ, it supports detox through sweat, releasing heat and waste, lightening the body from within. Your skin is a protective shield between the inner and outer world, as we also discuss in pillar 6.

Beyond these essential functions, your skin reflects what's going on inside. In *Āyurveda*, glowing skin isn't the goal, it's a natural outcome of inner balance, especially of *pittā doṣa*. When digestion, hormones and emotions are in harmony, the subtle glow of *tejas* (essence of *pittā*) naturally shine through.

If *Āyurveda* has taught me one thing, it's this: your skin doesn't just reflect what you put on it, it reflects what you put *in* your body. I witnessed this first-hand during a particularly stressful time in my mid-30s. My skin became reactive and dull, and no amount of topical care helped. The shift came only when I changed how I ate, managed the stress, added *rasāyana* herbs and, most importantly, prioritised sleep. Slowly, my inner glow returned.

Āyurveda recognises our skin, hair, nails and teeth as extensions of the quality of our *dhātus* (seven body tissues – *see also* pp. 45–6). When we deeply nourish our *dhātus*, especially *rasa* (plasma), *rakta* (blood) and *māṃsa* (muscle), which are closely linked to skin health, we not only support internal health but visibly slow down signs of ageing in our skin.

Just as our skin is linked to plasma, muscle and blood, our hair is linked to the quality of our bones (***asthi***), which are made mostly of collagen and minerals. So as bone mass declines, so too does hair strength and shine. That's why the guidance in chapters 3 and 5 and in pillar 1 is so important for our skin, too.

As we age, collagen production (the protein that gives skin its elasticity) naturally declines and studies show that in women, up to 30 per cent of the skin's collagen can be lost within the first five years after menopause. The skin can become thinner, more sensitive and slower to heal. Research confirms this is due to the drop in oestrogen, which also impacts muscle and bone density.

Science agrees that while hormonal changes influence skin ageing, external factors play a major role too. Sun damage and poor diet both accelerate skin ageing. UV rays create free radical damage and break down collagen. Diets high in sugar speed up skin ageing through *glycation*, a process that stiffens collagen fibres and makes them more prone to damage.

But there's good news. Early morning sunlight supports your hormonal health and circadian rhythm (as we explored in pillar 1), and well-loved rituals for skin, hair and nails can help us both look *and* feel good. Still, no cream compares to the glow that comes from a good night's sleep, a nourishing meal or the subtle confidence that builds when you care for yourself, deeply and daily. Let's explore pro-ageing ways to support your skin, starting with food.

Eat your skincare

Overleaf are some of my favourite everyday skin-loving foods that don't just support healthy skin but nourish you from the inside out.

Food	Why it's good for your skin
Ghee	An elixir that supports tissue repair, digestive harmony and *ojas*, helping sustain soft, resilient skin and lasting tissue vitality
Amalaki	Rich in vitamin C and antioxidants, *amalaki* stimulates collagen and tissue repair. It is a classic *rasāyana* for youthful skin (*see also* pp. 144–5)
Soaked almonds	Almonds contain vitamin E, healthy fats and protein, keeping skin hydrated and muscles strong for lifelong vitality
Mung dal	Easy to digest, mung dal is a source of amino acids and nutrients that supports clear skin, lean muscle and steady energy as we age
Pomegranate	Astringent and antioxidant-rich; purifies blood and helps to maintain firm, elastic skin through the years
Dates	Sweet, grounding and *bṛṃhaṇa* (nourishing), dates gently restore energy and strength, aiding recovery and sustaining resilience throughout life
Leafy greens	Rich in chlorophyll and nutrients, leafy greens detoxify, reduce inflammation and support lasting skin health
Carrots	High in beta-carotene and antioxidants, they protect skin, muscles, blood, vision and brighten skin tone
Beetroot	Beetroot boosts circulation, oxygenates tissues and promotes natural skin glow as we age
Sesame seeds	Mineral-rich (calcium, zinc, iron), sesame seeds strengthen bones, skin and connective tissue – foundational for longevity

Table 9.2 Skin-nourishing foods

What's in my radiance toolkit?

Now I won't claim to be a 'skincare' or 'beauty expert' because for me less has always been more and I truly believe in the power of radiance from within that is embedded in prevention and protection. Instead, let me share what my simple *Āyurvedic* skincare routine looks like on the days when I am feeling rather indulgent.

I start with gentle cleansing using rose water, which is great for its hydrating, astringent and soothing properties. Once a fortnight, I opt for a light and gentle Fuller's earth face pack (*Multani mitti*), mixed with rose water, turmeric or saffron and a few drops of oil. This natural clay purifies, tightens and brightens my skin, leaving me feeling refreshed and renewed.

I'm not exaggerating when I say I had my first professional facial in my late 40s, the much-talked-about HydraFacial. It was undeniably luxurious and left my skin feeling refreshed, but more than that, it reminded me how little time I'd given to skincare over the years. That experience was a turning point: I promised myself to create more space for pampering self-care, even if it's just for myself at home. Caring for your skin is a ritual of self-love – a way to honour the deeper layers of your being.

One of the most ancient and beloved *Āyurvedic* skincare practices is *ubṭana*. A blend of herbs, grain flours (like chickpea, barley or rice) and natural powders (such as sandalwood, turmeric or clay), it is traditionally used as a mask or scrub for the body and face to cleanse, exfoliate and bring out your inner glow. The combinations are endless and can be easily tailored to your skin's needs. Here are two simple DIY recipes I love for the face, with ingredients that are usually finer in texture than those used for the body:

Pro-ageing skin-exfoliating *ubṭana*

Ingredients:

- 1 tbsp chickpea flour (exfoliant and brightening)
- 1 tbsp ground oats or fine rice flour (gentle exfoliant)
- ¼ tsp turmeric (antibacterial and anti-inflammatory)
- 1 tsp raw honey (brightening and antibacterial)
- a few drops of milk, rose water or plain water, to make a spreadable paste (not too wet)
- Optional: neem, orange peel, sandalwood, musta, manjistha, ground almond

→

Method:

1. Mix all the ingredients to form a smooth, slightly thick paste.
2. Gently apply the paste to your damp face and neck, avoiding the eye area.
3. Leave on for five to 10 minutes, then wet your hands and gently massage in circular motions and scrub off for one minute.
4. Rinse off with lukewarm water and pat dry. Follow with a light face oil.

How to use:

Use once a week, preferably in the morning, to lift dullness and remove impurities.

Pro-ageing brightening face mask

Ingredients:

- 1 tsp *Multani mitti* (Fuller's earth) (deep cleansing and skin-firming)
- ½ tsp aloe vera gel (soothing and hydrating)
- pinch of saffron strands, soaked in 1 tsp warm milk for 10–15 minutes
- ½ tsp liquorice (*yaṣṭimadhu*) powder (for glow and pigmentation support)
- 1 tsp rose water (for oily/*pittā* skin) or milk (for dry/*vāta* skin)
- Optional: rose powder, orange peel, sandalwood, *mañjiṣṭhā*, turmeric, ground almond, ghee, coconut or almond oil

Method:

1. Mix the *Multani mitti* with the aloe vera gel, saffron-infused milk, liquorice powder and rose water or additional milk to form a smooth thin paste.
2. Apply to your clean face and neck.
3. Leave on for about 10 minutes (don't let it dry completely if your skin is dry).
4. Rinse off gently with cool water.
5. Moisturise with a light facial oil, such as rosehip, *kumkumādī* or jojoba.

How to use:

Use once a week, especially when skin feels tired and dry. This is designed to hydrate, calm and enhance natural glow.

Night shift for your skin

We know that night-time is the most powerful time for healing and your skin is no exception. I see it as tucking your skin into bed as you cleanse away the day, calm inflammation, seal in some essential nourishment and protect the deeper skin tissue from depletion. In the evening, I nourish my skin with *kumkumādī* oil, rosehip oil, jojoba oil or vitamin E oil, depending on its needs. These oils, rich in antioxidants and nutrients, promote radiance, repair damage and rejuvenate my skin. Just a few drops massaged in help the oils absorb more deeply and encourages healthy circulation.

I sometimes (not nearly as often as I know I should) incorporate a deeper facial massage with tools like the *kansa* wand, *gua sha* tool, facial cups or a jade roller. The *kansa* wand, rooted in *Āyurvedic* tradition, balances *doṣas,* improves circulation and eases tension, while the jade roller cools, depuffs and revitalises, transforming my skincare routine into a meditative ritual – check Resources, pp. 271–2 for *kansa* tools.

A new rule to live by: Don't put it on your skin, if you won't put it in your mouth!

While we may be conscious of staying hydrated, having nutrient-rich foods, healthy fats and essential vitamins and minerals in our diet, are we equally attentive to what we apply to our skin? A beautiful example of this is *Śatadhauta Ghṛta* – ghee washed 100 times until it becomes uniquely light, cooling and suitable for use as a nourishing skin moisturiser. If it's not edible, then don't feed it to your skin – after all, it's your biggest, most absorbent organ!

Āyurvedic face massage

There will always be the next new trend, from laser to stem cell therapy, all promising youthful, glowing skin. While many of these innovations have brought remarkable results, there's something healing about returning to time-tested traditions. *Āyurvedic* face massage is one of those gentle and deeply nourishing rituals, supporting the skin's natural ability to repair and renew.

While classical texts don't mention 'face yoga', facial massage is a longstanding part of *Āyurvedic* beauty and self-care. In my clinic, I work with *marma* points, activating the vital energy points using either a *kansa* wand or the fingertips to release tension, boost circulation and awaken a natural inner glow.

This gentle practice supports healthy microcirculation, delivering oxygen and nutrients to the skin while helping to detoxity and ease oxidative stress - a key factor in ageing.

It also encourages lymphatic flow, reduces puffiness and softens tension that can lead to fine lines. Over time, it helps maintain collagen and elastin production, keeping your skin firm and supple. Nourishing oils like the ones mentioned boost hydration and protection.

Pro-ageing facial *marma* ritual

Figure 9.1 below is a guide to gently massaging facial *marma* points, supporting circulation, skin health and overall vitality. Just two to five minutes of this loving ritual can leave your skin glowing and your nervous system grounded.

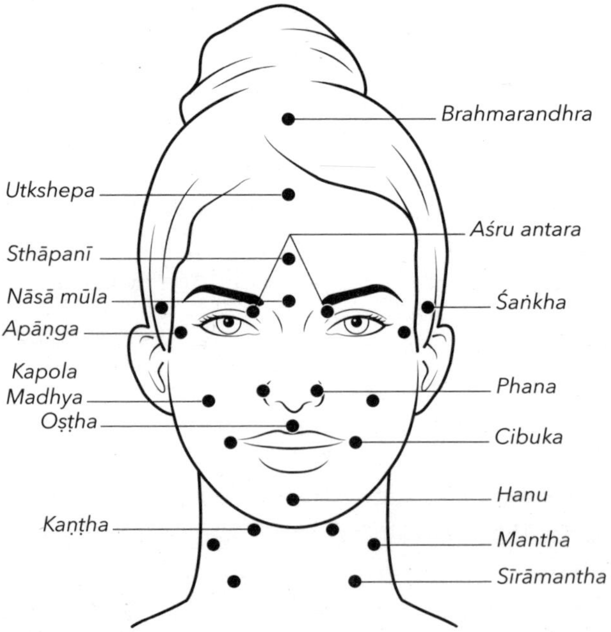

Figure 9.1 A map of the *marma* points (adapted from the teaching presented by Dr Vasant Lad - Marma Points of Āyurveda)

Here is how you can work through them:

1. Warm a few drops of a suitable face oil between your palms.
2. Start at the centre of your brow, gently circling the forehead (between the eyebrows) to calm the mind.
3. Move to the temples with small, soothing circles.
4. Using your ring fingers, lightly sweep under the eyes from the inner to the outer corners to ease puffiness.
5. Massage the cheeks and jaw with upward and outward strokes (a *kansa* wand works well too), then soften around the mouth with gentle circles.
6. Finish with light downward strokes from the jaw to the collarbone, to encourage lymph flow.

Heat v cold therapy

Āyurveda has always favoured treating with warmth over cold. Why? Because heat supports circulation, digestion and the flow of *prāṇa*. Cold, on the other hand, can constrict, slow things down and create stagnation in the body and mind – especially for women. It's especially aggravating for *vāta*, the *doṣa* most sensitive to imbalance, especially as we mature. Sorry to bear bad news, cold plunge enthusiasts!

In 2024, I experienced a traditional Russian Banya, an intense sauna-style heat ritual followed by an invigorating cold-water dousing and a cold plunge. My body went into severe shock: my heart started racing, my breath felt trapped and I couldn't shake the anxiety for hours after. My system felt like it had been assaulted, not energised. That was a clear message from my body that I need warmth, not shock therapy or extreme heat and cold in quick succession. Not all trends are nourishing for all body types, but if you're still game for cold-water practices, it works best when you build your tolerance slowly to prevent a 'cold shock' response.

Gentle treatments in *Āyurveda* with warm herbal oils and steam don't just warm the skin, they penetrate deep into the tissues, loosen toxins and create flow where there's stagnation. *Āyurveda* →

uses therapies that induce sweating, such as ***Svedana*** (herbal steam treatment) to mobilise and eliminate toxins, restore *doṣa* balance and support overall health. Modern sauna and steam practices echo this wisdom, thankfully.

Natural deodorants

In *Āyurveda*, sweating is recognised as a vital detox pathway, a natural process that helps regulate body temperature, maintain skin moisture and excrete water-soluble toxins through the skin.

Blocking the body's natural ability to sweat with antiperspirants, especially under the arms, may not be ideal. Some studies suggest that aluminium salts in antiperspirants can be absorbed through the skin, and show oestrogen-like activity in laboratory models, although the National Cancer Institute states that current human studies do not support a link to breast cancer – so for now, the jury is out.

Opting for natural deodorants that allow your body to sweat while neutralising bad odour can support your body's natural detoxification processes and lymphatic health. You can even opt for a simple coconut oil or the mineral alum (*fitkari*) – used for centuries in *Āyurvedic* and Unani medicine, gently supporting skin health with its antibacterial, antiseptic and astringent properties, especially where *pittā* and *kapha* imbalances (sweating, body odour) prevail.

Pro-ageing skin ritual

To combat the damaging effects of air pollution, now recognised as a major accelerator of ageing, I turn to *abhyanga*, a ritual of self-massage with warm herbal oils. This grounding practice nourishes the skin, supports gentle detoxification, encourages lymphatic flow and brings hydration to the deeper tissues. It also helps calm *vāta doṣa*, which when elevated, can lead to dryness, depletion and premature ageing.

A few mindful minutes of oiling your body (also known as *snehana*) with strokes up and down the limbs and around the joints before a shower can be a restorative act of self-care. During seasonal transitions like spring, when heaviness, sluggishness or *āma* are common, you can also do *garśana* (dry body brushing) to invigorate and stimulate the body. While Cleopatra may have bathed in milk for its nourishing and rejuvenation benefits, you too can indulge in the ritual of a warm bath after your *abhyanga* – add herbs, essential oils or even milk-based decoctions for the god/goddess in you.

Āyurvedic hair health

From my own experience with hair thinning after a period of intense stress, I've learned that it doesn't happen overnight, and neither does healing. It often begins through stress, nutritional gaps or imbalances that affect the body long before anything shows up on the scalp. And once it does, recovery takes time. Consistent care, inside and out, makes all the difference, even when results aren't immediate. Trust that your efforts are working. Focus on nourishment first and then bring in gentle haircare rituals. Let's look at inner support before moving to the outer steps.

Nourishment from within

The modern view is that hair is made of keratin, a protein, so a protein-rich diet is favoured. Nutrients like iron, vitamin D and healthy fats (*see* p. 113) help keep hair follicles healthy and reduce shedding.

Āyurveda goes deeper. Hair (*keśa*) is considered a *mala*, a by-product of *asthi dhātu* (bone tissue). Strong, healthy hair reflects strong, nourished bones. So, the root of hair health lies in building robust inner tissues, not just topical care.

Hormonal shifts, stress and lifestyle choices all impact hair health. When your core system is depleted or dry, your body triages its nourishment to vital tissues first, leaving hair, skin and nails more vulnerable – often the first signs of deeper imbalances.

Support for bone (hair) health is found through foods such as lentils, leafy greens, finger millet, nuts, seeds (especially sesame) and easily digestible dairy like warm milk, ghee, buttermilk or fresh paneer (if suitable) and animal proteins. If you're prone to sluggish digestion or congestion, go easy on heavier dairy like yoghurt. And don't overlook hydration and sunlight. Bones are linked to *vāta*, which is dry by nature, and internal dryness is often reflected as dryness in the hair, skin and nails. So, while hair may be made of protein, true radiance begins within – with strong digestion and *dhātu* formation (*see* chapter 3).

External haircare and *Āyurvedic* practices

While food builds from within, external rituals can support the process. Regular hair oiling is a time-tested *Āyurvedic* practice that strengthens hair, nourishes the scalp and calms the nervous system. Oils like *amalaki, brahmi, bṛṅgarāja, kalonji* (black seed), *bṛṅgādi* (a traditional blend of *Āyurvedic* oils), *eranda* (castor), sesame (black and white) and coconut are especially good for soothing the scalp, nourishing hair, reducing hair fall and minimising premature greying.

Protect your hair like you would your skin. Limit heat styling, avoid harsh sun exposure and use gentle, natural cleansers that don't strip away your scalp's natural oils. Trim it regularly to keep the ends healthy, and don't buy into the hype of miracle hair products.

Pro-ageing hair ritual

One of my favourite pro-ageing hair rituals is a soothing scalp massage. It boosts blood flow to the follicles, helping to deliver nutrients and supporting healthy growth. I slightly warm one of the oils mentioned and gently massage it in with my fingertips, then use my *kansa* comb to glide over the scalp in long strokes from front to back. The *kansa* alloy (copper and tin) is known to help balance pH, reduce heat and inflammation and subtly detoxify the scalp while improving circulation (*see* Resources, pp. 271–2, for *kansa* tools). This simple and soothing ritual helps relax the nervous system, stimulate the scalp and encourage better sleep and a calmer mind – all welcome side effects.

Is your environment healthful or harmful?

Our environment has a detrimental influence on the quality of our lives and how we age – physically, emotionally and energetically. It's not just the air we breathe or the water we drink: it's the social fabric we live in, our daily routines, the energy of our home and workspaces, the climate and even the healthcare systems we rely on.

Does your environment uplift or drain you? Creating a health-supportive atmosphere doesn't need to mean big changes – sometimes it begins with noticing what no longer serves you and making space for what does.

Our bodies are increasingly exposed to environmental toxins, polluted air, pesticide-laced food and plastics in everything, from packaging to cookware. In *Āyurveda*, these external toxins may act like *garaviṣa*: slow-acting, unnatural poisons that slowly build up over time and may trigger issues like allergies, infections and chronic disease.

The environmental impact on ageing

Whether we look back at the time when Vedic scriptures were documented or even compared to our grandparents' time, we now live in a radically different world. Pollution, urbanisation, deforestation, GMO farming, excess UV radiation and the overuse of chemicals have intensified oxidative stress, a key driver of premature ageing. The signs show up on the surface as dullness, dryness or fine lines, but below the surface, environmental stress disrupts cellular repair, fuels inflammation and impacts mental well-being and gut health – all detrimental to the way we age.

We're not just ageing due to time, but from the seemingly subtle toxic burden. Even the basic elements of life such as food, water and air are compromised in a way that our ancestors never had to contend with. Industrial agriculture has depleted our soil, leaving food less nutrient-rich. Additives, pesticides, microplastics, heavy metals and endocrine disruptors like BPA accumulate in the body, wearing down our natural resilience. I believe it's our shared responsibility to stay aware, so we can collectively resist what harms us, while restoring and protecting what sustains us.

Detox to make space in your body

It's no wonder we're seeing rising rates of chronic illness, hormonal imbalance and compromised vitality, even in the young. Our bodies were never meant to cope with this level of toxic exposure. And yet, we've normalised their symptoms and rush to 'fix' them without addressing the real drivers of the imbalance.

To truly heal, we must clear the clutter – physically, mentally, emotionally and environmentally. *Āyurveda* teaches that having clarity, lightness and vitality are not privileges but what's left when we remove what doesn't belong.

The invisible load of modern life

Sadly, it doesn't stop there. We have the new digital world – a world I value and embrace, but not without awareness. Our environment therefore isn't just physical, it's now digital too. Rapid advancement in technology, artificial intelligence (AI) and virtual reality (VR) is reshaping our biology in ways we don't yet fully understand for the long term. Constant virtual connectivity and screen exposure affect our nervous system, sleep, focus, mood and even our hormones and cellular balance. These shifts may not be visible (yet), but they are no less real and can influence how we age. As humans, the challenge is to be able to discern between technology as a tool and a technological takeover!

Here's how you can be more mindfully protective against digital and electromagnetic field (EMF) radiation:

- **Limit screen time** to minimise exposure to blue light, especially before bed.
- **Use blue-light-blocking glasses** to protect your eyes from digital strain.
- **Keep phones and laptops away from your body!** No more pockets, bra straps or laptops on your lap – the irony!
- **Use a speaker or headphones** when speaking on the phone rather than holding it to your ear.
- **Switch your phone to flight mode** before you sleep and keep it away from your bed.
- **Avoid wearing electronics to bed** (yes, even trackers and smartwatches). The Oura Ring, however, is reported to have very low electromagnetic field (EMF) exposure, if you must.
- **Minimise use of microwaves and air fryers** as they emit low-level EMF. Be intentional with safe, non-toxic cooking utensils and cookware.

We must question whether certain technologies and modern-day conveniences actually set us back when it comes to our health.

Taking a stand for vitality

Environmental stressors may feel beyond our control, but that doesn't mean we're powerless.

The good news? Small, mindful choices matter and can even be protective. By developing a conscious relationship with our environment, we can mitigate its impacts and support a truly pro-ageing way of living.

So, are you ready to be a disruptor? To choose calm in a chaotic world, and vitality over convenience? If so, read on ...

Pro-ageing environmental protection tips

- **Prioritise local, organic, seasonal and non-GMO**, antioxidant-rich foods to reduce exposure to toxins and support a healthy gut microbiome.
- **Drink plenty of clean, mineral-rich water**, such as naturally sourced spring water, to flush out toxins, maintain skin hydration and support cellular repair.
- **Opt for *Āyurvedic* or natural skincare products** free from harmful chemicals to nourish and protect the skin barrier. Read the labels of all your products, including toothpaste, deodorants and lip balms. You should recognise the ingredients. Avoid perfume and cologne and switch to natural essential oils. This was a subtle and cost-effective game changer for me, not to mention the fun you can have while creating your own blends.
- **Maintain proper ventilation in your home** by using air purifiers and increasing the number of houseplants such as snake plants, aloe vera or peace lilies to reduce exposure to pollutants in your living space (or at least lift your mood)!
- **Grow your own** or choose products from regenerative farming practices and support sustainable living by reducing waste and reusing and recycling. Give back by planting trees - evergreen hedges are a fabulous way to surround your home.
- **Use natural and eco-friendly house-cleaning solutions** and pest control and avoid artificial plug-in scents in your home/car to minimise synthetic chemicals. Opt for beeswax or soy candles made with essential oils or essential oil diffusers instead of cheap paraffin candles.

- **Drive less, walk and bike more**, or use public transport, where possible, to reduce pollution exposure while contributing to environmental sustainability. Avoid the main roads, where pollution exposure is much higher.

The sunscreen debate

Two decades of sailing trips and high sun exposure had gotten me into a frenzy about sun protection. I often find myself asking if we are protecting our skin or are we actually blocking something essential? Sunscreens, especially synthetic ones, were certainly not a part of daily life for my ancestors. Today, many people are applying them liberally, despite finding ourselves in an epidemic of vitamin D deficiency. Could it be the perfect example of a self-generated paradox?

Āyurveda, as always, takes a more nuanced view. The sun is not the enemy. It's the source of life and energy, crucial for immunity, mood and metabolism. The problem is the overexposure at the wrong time. Early morning sunlight is considered *bālya* (strengthening), especially for bone and hormone health. Stay in the shade or covered during the harsh *pittā* hours of 10 a.m. to 2 p.m. when the sun is most intense, not lathered in tanning oil, cooking yourself on the French Riviera.

Our skin is incredibly absorbent, especially when the pores are open from heat or sweating, so we must question what we're absorbing. Many conventional sunscreens and sprays contain endocrine-disrupting chemicals such as oxybenzone (benzophenone-3) and octinoxate (ethylhexyl methoxycinnamate). These have raised health concerns for both human health and marine ecosystems. A growing number of regions, including Hawaii and Palau, have banned sunscreens containing these chemicals in favour of mineral sunscreens – a nudge for us to choose better!

Āyurvedic texts don't speak of 'sunscreen' as we know them today, but they do suggest natural protective ingredients such as cooling herbs and oils like sandalwood, *mañjiṣṭhā*, liquorice, coconut oil and aloe vera, calming the skin stressed by heat and light exposure.

→

Modern research continues to explore these botanicals for their anti-inflammatory and antioxidant properties and their potential role in skin protection, which calm *pittā* and soothe UV-induced inflammation. These also double up as ingredients for deodorants.

Be like the iconic Audrey Hepburn – go for a wide-brimmed hat and a head scarf! Simply avoiding being outdoors during peak sun hours is still one of the wisest forms of protection today and no doubt for years to come.

Pillar 5

The luminous mind

'If the food is pure, the mind is pure. If the mind is pure, the memory is strong and steady.'

Chāndogya Upaniṣad

Age is an attitude! *Mens sana in corpore sano* means 'a healthy mind in a healthy body'. This echoes *Āyurveda's* belief in the constant dialogue between the mind and body, shaping each other's health and energy. While modern science emphasises neuroplasticity and cognitive stimulation to keep the brain healthy, *Āyurveda* focuses on balancing the three mental qualities, called *guṇas,* through ***Sattvavajaya*** (mastery of the mind). Here, the aim is to cultivate resilience and peace so that we can unlock a youthful, vibrant mind at any stage of life.

Just as the body needs cleansing in preparation for rejuvenation (as discussed in chapter 5), the mind too requires its own kind of clearing, which we explore in this pillar. Just like emptying the trash can on your computer helps it to function better, mental decluttering creates space for your mind to work more efficiently. This space helps cultivate the clarity, calm and resilience that keeps the mind youthful and the brain healthy.

So, what are the secrets for a youthful brain? This will be our focus in this pillar as we explore:

- The three *guṇas* – *sattva, rajas* and *tamas* – and how they shape clarity and balance
- *Prāṇa* as the subtle force of life, with two simple practices to regulate and renew it
- How to harness the power of words: mantras, affirmations and the inner stories that influence body and mind

- Ways to build mental resilience through study, reflection, creativity and connection with nature
- The healing effects of stillness through silence, time in nature and meditation such as ***trāṭaka*** and '***So Hum***'
- Shifting the mindset of ageing through gratitude and acceptance

बन्धुरात्मात्मनस्तस्य येनात्मैवात्मना जितः |
अनात्मनस्तु शत्रुत्वे वर्तेतात्मैव शत्रुवत् ||

Bandhur ātmātmanas tasya yenātmaivātmanā jitaḥ |
Anātmanas tu śatrutve vartetātmaiva śatruvat ||

'For him who has conquered the mind, the mind is the best of friends; but for one who has failed to do so, his very mind works like an enemy.'

Bhagavad Gītā, 6:6

Guṇas – the three mental qualities

In a state of constant flux, the *guṇas* (the mind's qualities) – *sattva*, *rajas* and *tamas* – influence our thoughts, actions and emotions, and subsequently impact healthspan and longevity. Let's explore each one here …

Sattva – cultivate clarity and balance

Sattva is the quality of lightness, tranquillity, clarity, purity, compassion, wisdom and joy. When *sattva* is strong within us, we feel grounded, content and steady. We're less reactive and more resilient to stress, one of the primary drivers of premature ageing and disease.

A *sattvic* mind supports clear thinking and mental agility. It helps reduce oxidative stress and nourishes the tissues, supports mental acuity and protects the brain from cognitive decline well into our later years.

So how do we cultivate *sattva* in daily life?

Vedic wisdom encourages using practices that soothe and elevate our spirit. Simple, consistent rituals like meditation, such as *Vipassanā*, Transcendental Meditation (TM) or silent sitting can do wonders. Living with intention, choosing kindness, speaking truthfully and practising non-violence (*ahiṃsā*) create an inner environment where *sattva* flourishes. Gratitude and time spent in nature also regulate our nervous system by cultivating *sattva*. And let's not forget that fresh, light *sattvic* foods, such as fruits, vegetables, whole grains, milk, ghee and herbs, also cultivate *sattva*.

Rajas: the energy of activity and restlessness

Rajas is the mind quality that gets things moving. It fuels our passion, ambition and courage. It's what motivates us to set goals, exercise, create and pursue meaningful change. In the right dose, *rajas* drives purposeful action when guided by awareness. But when it intensifies, it can leave us feeling restless, irritable or burnt out. Too many deadlines, too much screen time, stimulants or even trying to constantly improve ourselves can push the nervous system into a frenzy. This kind of chronic overstimulation wears us down, disturbing sleep and speeding up ageing over time.

So how do we balance *rajas* in daily life?

To bring *rajas* into balance, lean into rest and rhythm. Regular meals, consistent sleep and gentle movement help regulate the inner unrest. Practices like yoga, tai chi or simply slowing down your mornings can soften and settle excess *rajas*. Choose calming and grounding foods and cut back on stimulants like caffeine, alcohol, spicy foods and fried foods to steady the mind.

Tamas: the force of rest and inertia

Tamas is the mind quality of stillness, stability and rest. It's the energy that allows deep sleep, restoration and renewal - all essential for vitality and longevity. *Tamas* helps us slow down, restore and heal. Without it, there'd be no true rest or recovery.

But when *tamas* slips into excess, we can start to feel heavy, dull and lethargic. You might notice yourself feeling sluggish, unmotivated, mentally foggy or emotionally low. If it lingers, it can lead to more serious imbalances like isolation, depression or a sense of feeling stuck in self-comparison and regret, all of which affect long-term health and clarity.

So how do we lighten *tamas* in daily life?

The goal isn't to get rid of *tamas*, but to keep it in check. If you feel stuck or foggy, gently activate your mind and body. Read something that inspires you, learn a new skill, get sunlight exposure, move regularly and eat lighter, more *prāna*-rich foods. Even small shifts can spark clarity and renewal. By reducing heavy, stale or processed foods and choosing fresh, vibrant meals you can lift that mental dullness.

The aim is to cultivate more *sattva*, balance *rajas*, and minimise *tamas*, restoring inner balance. Each time we 'add in' a bit more *sattva* through meditation, mantra and *sattvic* food, we naturally regulate *rajas* and *tamas*.

Fuel for brain nourishment

Medhya rasāyanas, or brain-supporting rejuvenatives, includes both food, as explored in pillar 2, and herbs like *brahmi*, *gotu kola* and *aśvagandhā* - *see* pillar 3. Together they nurture mental clarity, support cognitive rejuvenation and sustain vitality for pro-ageing. Beyond nourishment and herbs, mental well-being rests on the upkeep of a *sattvic* mind, steered by the subtle life force within - *prāṇa*.

No *prāṇa*? No life!

As we explored in chapter 3, *prāṇa* is the subtle but essential energy that permeates life into every cell, organ and thought. Without *prāṇa*, there is no vitality, no movement, no clarity, no capacity to heal and no life, for that matter. *Prāṇa* is the exact force that separates life from death, and breath is our most malleable way to regulate *prāṇa*. Yet most of us move through our days using only a fraction of our breath's potential, disconnected from tapping into this vital energy.

How *prāṇa* moves through us

Oxygen nourishes our cells, fuels mitochondrial energy and keeps every organ and tissue alive. But, with each inhale, we take in more than oxygen - we draw in *prāṇa*. *Prāṇa* moves more subtly, flowing through the body's gross *and* subtle channels to sustain physical, mental and emotional balance. The breath is the vehicle that bridges our inner worlds.

Science echoes the same message: every cell needs oxygen to survive. Without it, even for a few minutes, irreversible damage can occur. Because the body doesn't store oxygen, we must keep supplying it through the breath. But stress, shallow breathing and tension can reduce that flow, affecting everything from mental clarity to immune strength. Did you know that it is very common to unconsciously hold our breath while we are scrolling? Something referred to as screen apnea!

Prāṇa flows through three main *nādīs* (energy channels): *iḍā* (left side, cooling lunar energy), *piṅgalā* (right side, activating solar energy) and *suṣumṇā* (the central *nādī*), which begin at the base of the spine (*mūlādhāra*) and rise to the crown (*sahasrāra*) and are considered in yoga as the pathways of spiritual awakening. These three key channels weave through the seven *chakras* (energy centres), which, interestingly, correlate with our endocrine glands at each intersection. Each gland produces hormones, acting as the body's master regulators for growth, metabolism, reproduction, stress-response, mood and overall balance. Coincidence? I think not! When the breath is shallow or restricted, these channels constrict and *prāṇa* can't flow freely. Over time, this can deplete nourishment to the *dhātus* (body tissues) and mind (*manas*).

On average, a person breathes about 18 times per minute. Take a moment to count your natural breaths per minute. Animals that breathe quickly, like monkeys (around 25 breaths per minute), tend to live shorter lives - 25 years, while slow-breathing creatures such as tortoises can live for over a century (around four breaths per minute). The *Hatha Yoga Pradipika* teaches that slow breathing increases vitality and strengthens the heart, elongating the lifespan, a principle validated by numerous research studies.

The good news is that the breath is something we can learn to direct. *Prāṇāyāma*, the yogic practice of conscious breathing and energy regulation, helps increase the flow of oxygen and *prāṇa* throughout the body. It supports the tissues, regulates the nervous system and brings balance across body and mind. This isn't just a mind-calming ritual, it's a full body energy reset.

I've had consistent breath practice for years, and even on the busiest mornings, just a few minutes of deep breathing helps me feel clearer, more grounded and better able to move through my day. Start by simply becoming more aware of your breath as you walk or do house chores. Let's explore two simple but deeply effective breathing practices that you can add to your morning routine to bring calmness to the mind by enhancing *sattva* and regulated flow of *prāṇa* to your entire system.

Morning channel cleanser – *Nādī Śodhana*

Nādī Śodhana, or alternate nostril breathing, is one of my favourite ways to start the day. It's a gentle practice that soothes the mind and regulates the nervous system, helping *prāṇa* flow more freely through the subtle energy channels.

Prāṇayama is not just 'breathing exercises', it is the practice of guiding life force into the deeper tissues, enhancing *ojas* and gently clearing blockages in the subtle *nādīs*. The lunar channel, *iḍā*, is cooling and connected to the right brain and parasympathetic system. *Piṅgalā*, the solar channel, is activating and linked with the left brain and sympathetic system. When there is harmony between *iḍā* and *piṅgalā* it encourages energy to flow through *suṣumṇā*, supporting integration and spiritual awakening.

By softly alternating the breath between the nostrils, *Nādī Śodhana* nurtures balance between the left (the analytical) and right (the intuitive) brain, lunar and solar energies, and the body's stress response. This simple yet profound practice can ease anxiety, fatigue, mood swings and even high blood pressure, promoting emotional steadiness, softening extreme moods such as irritability, sadness, or restlessness over time.

You might be surprised how just a few minutes of steady, rhythmic breathing can clear the fog, calm the mind and create a sense of spaciousness. It's a beautiful ritual to begin the day, supporting both mental clarity and tissue vitality.

Nādī Śodhana

1. Practise in a quiet, well-ventilated space.
2. Sit comfortably with your spine upright and shoulders relaxed – try *Sukhāsana* (cross-legged), *Vajrāsana* (kneeling) or sitting on a chair.
3. Use your right thumb to close your right nostril, then inhale slowly and deeply through the left nostril without straining. (Advanced practice – hold the inhalation for a count of four.)
4. Close the left nostril with your ring finger, open the right nostril and exhale completely without straining. (Advanced practice – hold the exhalation for a count of four.)
5. Inhale slowly and deeply through the right nostril without straining, close it. (Advanced practice – hold the inhalation for a count of four.) Then exhale through the left nostril.
6. Repeat for five to 10 minutes.

Safety first: If you feel light-headed, return to natural breathing. Avoid breath retention (*kumbhaka*) unless guided by a qualified teacher, especially if you're pregnant or managing heart or blood pressure conditions.

Morning energiser: *Kapālabhāti*

Kapālabhāti, often called 'Skull Shining Breath', is an invigorating practice that clears mental fog and wakes up the entire body. Unlike the gentle rhythm of *Nādī Śodhana*, this one's energising – perfect for mornings, springtime or whenever you need a natural lift in energy.

It involves short, active, belly-powered exhalations, while the inhalations stay soft and passive. This rhythm stimulates circulation, floods fresh oxygen to the brain, leaving you feeling lighter and mentally alert.

Kapālabhāti stimulates *agni*, metabolism and supports the natural elimination pathways. Practised regularly, it nourishes all the tissues and brightens the mind, supporting vitality by flooding them both with *prāṇa*. It pairs beautifully with *Nādī Śodhana* to start your day both uplifted and grounded.

Kapālabhāti

1. Sit comfortably with your spine straight and shoulders relaxed – try *Sukhāsana* (cross-legged), *Vajrāsana* (kneeling) or sitting on a chair. It's best practised in morning *kapha* hours (6–10 a.m.).
2. Take a deep breath in and exhale fully.
3. Inhale to about 50 per cent capacity, then exhale strongly in short and sharp bursts through the nose, pulling your abdomen inwards with each exhalation. Let inhalations happen passively.
4. Do 20–30 strong exhalations, then take a few deep breaths and relax.
5. Gradually increase to three rounds of 20–30 exhalations.

Safety first: Avoid during pregnancy, or if you have high blood pressure, heart concerns or respiratory issues. If you feel dizzy or fatigued, stop and rest.

The power of words

Whether in conversation, self-talk or even our inner thoughts, our choice of words can powerfully influence the qualities of our mind (*guṇas*). This is because language is not just descriptive, it actively shapes how we perceive, feel and experience our own energy.

Negative self-talk can become slow self-destruction for our well-being. Our body cannot discern what is real and what is perceived, so it believes us regardless, just as it cannot distinguish actual stress from perceived stress. For example:

- A ***tamasic*** inner voice might sound like *I'm hopeless* or *Nothing will ever change*, breeding apathy and heaviness.

- ***Rajasic*** self-talk often fuels anger and restlessness – *I'm not doing enough* or *Why am I still behind?* – driving self-criticism and burnout.
- In contrast, ***sattvic*** self-talk is gentle, grounded and uplifting – *I'm learning* or *I trust the process*.

Why do our words matter in the context of ageing? Because the mind doesn't just age with the body, it shapes *how* we age. What we speak, chant or think directly influences our biochemistry, nervous system, emotional resilience and even how well our cells regenerate. *Rajasic* or *tamasic* mental patterns including chronic negative self-talk can activate physiological stress pathways – fuelling inflammation, disrupting cortisol rhythms and depleting our emotional reserves – processes widely discussed as relevant to accelerated ageing. In contrast, cultivating a more *sattvic* inner environment through conscious speech, mantras and affirming words can potentially enhance inner steadiness, joy and neuroplasticity by activating brain systems for reward and self-related processing.

This is why really listening to the language of my clients paints a thousand words outside of their presenting symptoms. Consciously choosing positive language can shift your mindset and open up new possibilities, so let's look at how you can begin to do this.

Change your narrative – change your trajectory

Table 10.1 overleaf contains some quick word swaps I find useful to help reframe my mindset towards acceptance, learning, growth, problem-solving and confidence.

Conscious speech and sacred sound are subtle forms of *rasāyana*, nourishing the mind and emotions. Just as negative daily dialogue adversely shapes the mind, Vedic chants and mantras can positively offer a reframe. Let's explore these as tools for cultivating *sattva*.

Limiting belief	Empowering reframe
I can't do this.	*I'm in a learning process.*
I always mess things up.	*I'm getting better with practice.*
This is too hard.	*It may feel challenging, but I am capable.*
I constantly make mistakes.	*I grow through the lessons.*
I'm not good enough.	*I'm enough just as I am.*
Everything always goes wrong.	*I adapt and keep improving through every hurdle.*
I don't deserve success.	*I am worthy of good things.*
I'm stuck.	*I'm exploring new possibilities.*

Table 10.1 How to reframe your mindset

Vedic chants and mantras

In the ancient Vedic tradition, mantras were considered to be vibrational tools meant to be experienced while working on the subtle layers of the self (our inner *kośas* – *see* p.68), not just accepted as religious recitations. Sages understood that sound could heal, harmonise and rewire the mind, long before neuroscience confirmed its effects. We are already beginning to see evidence that chanting ancient Vedic sounds helps to calm the nervous system, support mental clarity and positively influence brainwave activity.

Chanting mantras with intention – whether Vedic, Buddhist, Shamanic or affirmations you create yourself – can open space for healing, shift your vibration, dissolve internal resistance and cultivate *sattva*.

I invite you to discover healing through both words and sounds by consciously choosing words that are kind to your mind, especially through repetitive chants. Overleaf are a few Vedic mantras along with modern affirmations focused on vitality and longevity. Incorporate them into your daily routine by speaking them aloud or quietly reciting them during peaceful moments. Notice how they feel in your body and allow them to become seeds of transformation.

Mahā Mṛtyuñjaya Mantra (for healing and liberation from death)

This classic *shiva* mantra is often recited for longevity, to prevent suffering and premature death:

ॐ त्र्यम्बकं यजामहे सुगन्धिं पुष्टिवर्धनम् ।
उर्वारुकमिव बन्धनान्मृत्योर्मुक्षीय माऽमृतात्॥

Oṃ tryambakaṃ yajāmahe sugandhiṃ puṣṭi-vardhanam |
urvārukam iva bandhanān mṛtyor mukṣīya mā'mṛtāt ||

'We honour the one with three eyes, the fragrant nourisher who increases vitality. Like a ripe fruit released from its vine, may I be liberated from death but not from immortality.'

Ṛgveda, 7.59.12.

Gāyatrī Mantra (for wisdom and enlightenment)

The *Gāyatrī Mantra* is one of the most sacred and powerful mantras in the Vedic tradition, revered as a prayer for inner illumination, health and well-being. It's a call to the divine light of the radiant sun asking it to guide our thoughts and awaken the clarity within, which is why it's traditionally chanted at sunrise. It's a beautiful way to reconnect with your inner wisdom, feel more focused and align your energy with the rhythms of nature. Just a few moments with this mantra can bring calm and a sense of inner strength. Give it a try:

ॐ भूर् भुवः स्वः। तत् सवितुर्वरेण्यं ।
भर्गो देवस्य धीमहि धियो यो नः प्रचोदयात्॥

oṃ bhūr bhuvaḥ svaḥ | tat savitur vareṇyaṃ |
bhargo devasya dhīmahi | dhiyo yo naḥ pracodayāt ||

'We meditate on the sacred radiance of the divine Savitar. May he illuminate our minds.'

Ṛgveda, 3.62.10

Pāvamāna Mantra (for purification and immortality)

This mantra is another simple yet powerful chant for inner clarity and spiritual renewal. It's a gentle request for guidance from illusion to truth, from confusion to light, and from fear of death to a sense of timeless peace. Often used at the end of rituals, it helps us return to our centre, feeling lighter, clearer and more connected to something deeper within:

असतो मा सद्गमय। तमसो मा ज्योतिर्गमय। मृत्योर्मा अमृतं गमय।
ॐ शान्तिः शान्तिः शान्तिः॥

Asato mā sadgamaya, tamaso mā jyotirgamaya |
mṛtyor mā amṛtaṃ gamaya. Aum śāntiḥ, śāntiḥ, śāntiḥ ||

Lead me from the unreal to the real; lead me from darkness to light; lead me from death to immortality, Aum peace, peace, peace.
Bṛhadāraṇyaka Upanishad, 1.3.28

Modern-day affirmations

Not everyone will want to immerse into Vedic mantras, so here are a few modern-day affirmations that I hope will resonate as valuable alternatives:

- *I honour the inner wisdom of my body and trust its rhythm.*
- *Every breath renews my vitality and strengthens my spirit.*
- *I mature with grace, clarity and conscious joy.*
- *My radiance grows brighter with each passing year.*
- *I am intimately connected to nature, the cosmos and my deeper self.*
- *Healing flows through me like a steady, sacred river.*
- *I embrace time as a teacher, not an inhibitor.*

Mental radiance as we age

Longevity isn't just about clocking more years, it's about staying mentally sharp, curious and vibrant. And no matter what your stage of life, that journey starts today. As we mature, it's natural for our cognitive function to alter. Factors like poor sleep, hormonal changes, anxiety, low mood and even certain social habits can influence our mental clarity over time.

You might wonder how some people seem to stay mentally agile well into their later years. This is where the idea of 'cognitive reserve' comes in – our brain's capacity to adapt and stay functional over time despite change or decline. From an *Āyurvedic* perspective, this can be influenced by our *prakṛti* (our unique mind–body constitution). Modern research adds that an engaging education early in life, a fulfilling job, mentally stimulating hobbies and a generally healthy lifestyle all help build this reserve.

Thankfully, cognitive resilience isn't fixed: we can build and nurture it. *Āyurveda* encourages dietary and lifestyle practices, which we explore throughout this book, that nourish *ojas* (vital essence) and cultivate *sattva* to maintain, develop and strengthen cognitive resilience.

Aside from the *prāṇāyāma* practices and mantra recitations that we've explored so far, how else can we actively build our cognitive resilience?

To stay mentally sharp as we age, we must continue to engage our curiosity, through reading, self-inquiry, learning new things, connecting with nature and inviting newness. Just as your body thrives on movement, your mind thrives on stimulation, wonder and creative exploration. Let's learn more about these simple, meaningful and practical ways forward.

Use it before you lose it!

Building cognitive resilience (*manas-bala*) begins with showing up each day with curiosity and authenticity. It starts the moment we become aware – right now! When we engage our minds simply for the joy of learning, rather than pressure to perform, it becomes deeply fulfilling.

Whether it's picking up a new skill, learning a language, reading more often (as well as aloud) or even revisiting a pre-loved hobby, it all counts to promote neuroplasticity and maintain cognitive function. Try playing cards or board games, listening to a thought-provoking podcast like TED Talks, signing up for an online course or getting inspired by wandering through a gallery or museum. Swap screen time for soul time. Volunteer, get creative or relearn something with your children or grandchildren. Even choosing a retreat over a typical poolside holiday can refresh the mind in surprising ways. The key is to stay engaged with life and yourself through continued learning.

Stimulate your creative juices

When we stimulate the right side of our brain, we engage more with our artistic self – the part that's softer, more open, flexible and less judgemental. Modern research strongly links creativity and cognitive reserve, just as *Āyurveda* teaches that creativity arises from the clarity of *sattva* and also helps sustain it. Creative expression disrupts rigid patterns (*rajas* and *tamas*) and encourages more expansive, lateral thinking.

It's never too late to start or to try something new and when it comes to creativity, there is no right or wrong, just exploration and expression. In my clinic, I often meet clients who worry that they haven't found their direction in life (their *dharma*) but sometimes variety can be equally nourishing.

Getting your creative juices flowing can activate brain systems involved in reward and motivation and may support more positive perceptions of one's creative abilities. So, are you going to get doodling? Large population studies show that engaging in creative and mentally enriching activities can reduce the risk of cognitive decline and dementia.

So, what kind of artist lives dormant within you? You could explore writing, painting, playing a musical instrument, photography, pottery, acting, poetry or anything else that stirs inspiration. These activities spark neuroplasticity and strengthen emotional well-being. Creative problem-solving also engages the prefrontal brain systems that support flexible thinking and the evaluation of novel ideas.

The novelty of newness

'Insanity is doing the same thing over and over again and expecting different results.' Albert Einstein wasn't just being witty, he understood that novelty fires up the brain. Every time we do something unfamiliar, even just through imagination, we spark new neural pathways. That feeling of expansion when we dream/daydream or try something new? That's your brain lighting up, adapting and growing.

Research from the Blue Zones (*see also* p. 24) shows a common thread among long-living communities: a strong sense of purpose, play and lifelong curiosity, all of which contribute to emotional and physical resilience. Whether through hobbies, meaningful work or social connection, staying mentally flexible helps protect against cognitive decline.

Trying something new doesn't have to mean skydiving. It can be as simple as rearranging your furniture, taking a different route to work, trying a new spice, switching up your routines, trying a new class or listening to a music genre you'd usually skip. It's about gently nudging yourself out of the familiar.

In 2024, I hiked and ziplined through the jungles of Laos and stayed in an eco-friendly treehouse – absolutely exhilarating! I love to travel because it wakes something up in me – it is a version of *newness* for me. There's a richness in being immersed in new cultures, surrounded by nature and meeting people whose stories expand our own. It's stimulating, grounding and deeply human, reminding me how vast and connected the world truly is. I also joined a dinner arranged by an organisation, where six strangers are matched through an algorithm to share a meal, drinks, stories and ideas. It pushed me out of my comfort zone and into rich, meaningful conversations I would never have had otherwise. It was a brilliant reminder that growth often hides in unfamiliar places.

So, here's a gentle challenge: stay safe, but don't stay stuck. Shake things up – creatively, socially, mentally – and let your brain know you're still curious, still evolving.

Reading and self-inquiry

Sure, there's a time and place for a little Netflix, but if we're talking about building cognitive strength, that's not what's going to stretch and flex your neural pathways. Interestingly, studies on longevity have shown that reading books (not just skimming magazines or newspapers) can add up to two extra years to your life. A Yale study even found that reading for just three to four hours a week was linked with higher life expectancy. Why? Because reading is slower; it's immersive. It invites inquiry, imagination, emotional engagement and expansion of vocabulary and offers a broader lens on life beyond our own thoughts.

Svādhyāya, the practice of self-study and introspection rooted in Yogic and Vedic traditions, plays a profound role in promoting mental health and longevity. By encouraging self-reflection through meditation and journalling, and most importantly, reading sacred texts such as the *Bhagavad Gītā* and Upanishads, or modern self-development books, allows the reader to develop deeper introspection about life as well as feel expansive and limitless.

Therefore, regular *svādhyāya* may engage brain networks involved in self-related reflection and meaning-making. These types of contemplative practices are associated with approaches shown to support cognitive flexibility. It also gently steers us towards a sense of *dharma*, which both *Āyurveda* and now modern science recognise as integral to pro-ageing.

Embracing stillness

Real self-care often begins with the courage to say no, especially to the constant demands of others. Finding the right balance between social interaction and solo time is an art with a quest to cultivate *sattva*. Taking quiet moments to rest and reflect brings us into the present – the only moment that is truly real.

Embracing stillness can be simple – try journalling, reading, making art, lighting a candle, use a grounding essential oil or actively observing nature's surroundings. All these small acts create space for inner clarity. I love encouraging gratitude and reflection through curated journalling prompts as well as slowing things down by writing with your non-dominant hand. They become a vehicle for deeper self-inquiry through gentle challenge (*see* pillar 7).

Stillness can be nurtured through many of the practices we've already explored, like mantra chanting, visualisation and breathwork. Regular meditation has been shown to sharpen cognitive function, support neuroplasticity and ease the effects of stress on the mind and body.

As we learned in chapter 2, one of the most powerful rejuvenative practices in classical *Āyurveda* is *kuti praveśikā* (rejuvenation therapy during isolation in a hut). While I haven't done this in its classical form, I've had glimpses of its essence. In rural Mexico, I experienced a *temazcal*, a kind of traditional sweat lodge. Sitting in silence, completely alone, inside a low-ceiling, purpose-built clay dome, I felt an initial wave of discomfort and claustrophobia. But with time and a focus on the breath, the silence allowed me to soften, to notice my inner chatter.

Some years ago, my first 10-day *Vipassanā* silence retreat (a Buddhist meditation practice) similarly brought many challenges and revelations. The idea of being immersed in complete silence for 10 full days while detached from the outside world felt both daunting and deeply needed. No phones, no journals, not even a yoga mat. Just you and your mind. No communication with anyone except your own thoughts. I began to realise that we're not only constantly distracted by the noise around us, but more so by the noise within, the constant chatter inside the confines of our own shell. With nowhere to turn, the universe pushes you to resolve any challenges from within, and slowly, you begin to learn how to become your own best friend. When there is no place to escape, you have no choice but to surrender to the journey of self. It may sound intense, and at times it is, but the sensations, revelations and rewards are second to none. You come back into the world with a renewed sense of self, mentally resilient and with a whole new way of seeing life.

Of course, we don't all need to do something so extreme. What matters most is that we gently compound the benefits day by day through regular meditation and moments of silence. These days, I enjoy a healthy balance of time with friends, family and community, with solo time for silence, contemplation and deep restoration. Helping you to create more of this balance is what we will continue to explore in the rest of this pillar.

Inactivity is an activity: the power of silence

When was the last time you truly sat in silence – just you, your thoughts, your breath? No phone, no music, no book, no distractions? In our fast-paced, hyper-connected world, silence has become a rare and almost an uncomfortable experience, but in its absence, we lose something vital: the ability to hear our own inner voice.

→

In *Āyurveda* and Yogic traditions, ***mauna***, the observance of intentional silence, is revered as a powerful practice for mental clarity and emotional balance. Though it may seem like sitting and doing nothing, it's actually a conscious pause that nourishes the nervous system, calms mental chatter and helps us reconnect with ourselves.

How might life feel if we created more space for these quiet, healthful moments? Morning is one of the most potent times to practise *mauna*, when the world is still awakening and the mind is most receptive to clarity, calm and inner connection (*see also brahma muhūrta*, pp. 102–3).

Meditation for daily life

I'm not opposed to meditation apps at all. They're a wonderful gateway, offering short, guided sessions that can help ease stress, calm the mind and improve focus. After all, something is better than nothing. But traditional meditation practice is ultimately a path to deep transformation. It's about self-realisation, transcending the ego and connecting to higher states of consciousness. These practices often ask for more time and discipline, usually guided by a teacher, and lead us far beyond simple stress relief.

Whatever your entry point, my message is simple: meditation isn't just something you 'do' – it's a vehicle for remembering who you *are*. It's how we grow older *and* wiser. How we stay connected to something deeper, even while everything else keeps changing. Meditation has always been an anchor for me, especially in the process of writing this book.

Regular meditation has been shown to reduce psychological stress with Mindfulness-based programmes, producing measurable improvements in anxiety, depression and pain. Beyond the mind, meditation also supports physical health by lowering blood pressure, improving immune function and reducing inflammation. In older adults, regular mindfulness and breathing practices further improve sleep quality, reduce fatigue and depressive symptoms, and enhance overall well-being in older adults with moderate sleep disturbances. Meditation is associated with increased frontal theta activity (4–8Hz).

Could these states promote psychological conditions for introspection, reflection and changes in habitual thinking?

There are many traditional meditation practices to explore, each offering a unique path inwards. You might be drawn to ***dhyāna*** (yogic meditation), the silent stillness at the heart of classical yoga, or to mantra and *japa* meditation, where repetition brings focus to the mind. Practices like *Vipassanā* and *hṛdaya* meditation cultivate deep self-awareness, while *trātaka* (flame-gazing), *Nāda Yoga* (sound meditation) and ***likhita japa*** (meditative writing) offer more sensory or expressive approaches. *Kriyā Yoga* and *Yoga Nidrā* blend breath, awareness and energy flow, highlighting that meditation can be both still and dynamic.

Low energy, digital fatigue, brain fog, poor sleep, headaches, stiff neck? So many of us have been feeling the strain. Sometimes, what we need isn't more input, but a gentle way to reset. Let me share two of my favourite meditation practices with you. They're both powerful yet easy to practise, whether you're a beginner or a seasoned yogi.

Trātaka (flame-gazing meditation)

Meditation *is* medicine and lately I've been drawn back to *trātaka*, a beautifully simple practice that helps quieten the mind – something we all need now and then. *Trātaka*, a practice of steady gazing (typically on a naked flame), is especially beneficial for busy, *vāta*-type minds. It is one of the ***ṣaṭkarmas*** (cleansing techniques) described in the *Haṭha Yoga Pradīpikā*, used to purify the mind and sharpen concentration. You sit, gaze without blinking, and eventually the eyes naturally release water, which is like a subtle cleansing.

This practice is said to awaken the *ājñā chakra* (third eye), guiding our awareness inwards and helping us move from mental noise to deeper insight. It is believed to support the pineal gland, which helps regulate sleep and circadian rhythms. Even just a few minutes can ease tension, calm the nervous system and bring you back to your centre. It is best practised at dawn or dusk, in a quiet, darkened space, on an empty stomach.

How to practise:

1. Sit comfortably with your spine upright, shoulders relaxed; rest your hands on your knees – palms facing upwards. Add a *mudrā* (hand gesture), such as *gyan mudrā*, if you like.

→

2. Place a ghee lamp or candle at eye level, about an arm's length away.
3. Begin with closed eyes, then open them and gaze gently at the flame's centre without blinking, until your eyes water.
4. Close your eyes and continue to visualise the flame until the image fades.
5. Repeat as you feel called.

Safety note: Consult your practitioner if you suffer from eye health issues.

'So Hum' meditation

'So Hum' is an ancient Sanskrit mantra meaning 'I am that', symbolising the unity of self with universal consciousness. This meditation helps quieten the mind, deepen self-awareness and awaken a connection to your higher self.

If you are new to meditation, you can start this meditation practice with as little as five minutes and increase your time from there. The key is gentle repetition and openness to subtle shifts in awareness. I highly recommend learning Vedic meditation with an authentic spiritual guide.

1. Sit comfortably with a straight back and relaxed shoulders, hands resting in your lap. Close your eyes.
2. Take a few slow, deep breaths to settle your body and mind.
3. As you inhale slowly, silently say, *So*. As you exhale slowly, silently say, *Hum*.
4. Let the mantra flow naturally with your breath – there's no need to force or control it.
5. With each breath, allow your body to soften and your awareness to deepen, taking your attention towards the forehead, the heart or the navel centre.
6. When thoughts arise, gently notice them and return to your breath and the mantra, without judgement.
7. Continue for 15–20 minutes, letting the breath and mantra guide you into stillness.
8. To finish, stop repeating the mantra, take a few natural breaths, then rub your hands together and place them over your eyes before opening them.

The healing power of nature

If meditation feels daunting, simply begin by spending quiet time in nature: a gentle walk, sitting under a tree or just observing the moving clouds in the sky. Nature has a profoundly calming and grounding effect on the mind and body. In fact, research suggests that walking in natural environments may help reduce inflammation in the body – a key driver in ageing and chronic diseases like diabetes, Alzheimer's and heart disease. Studies also link time spent in green spaces with lower mortality rates and reduced risk of both physical and mental health conditions. Maybe this is why I cannot get enough of my daily walks in the woods – a chance to fully immerse my senses, smelling the earth, listening to the stream and birds, touching the trees.

From an *Āyurvedic* lens, reconnecting with the five elements (*pañca mahābhūtas* – earth, water, fire, air and space) restores balance within at the deepest level. We are a microcosm of the cosmos (***tat tvam asi***). Practices like earthing, forest bathing (*shinrin-yoku*) or simply immersing yourself in nature helps regulate the nervous system and awaken inner stillness.

Nature becomes a tender teacher. Through her rhythms and cycles, we're inspired to slow down, to observe, to be patient. She shows us how to release what no longer serves and fearlessly renew ourselves, again and again.

Creating mindset shifts for pro-ageing

To wrap up this pillar, consider how our mindset can shape how we age, from shifting our age narrative, adopting gratitude as an attitude and trusting our inner wisdom to achieve lasting results.

Reframing the narrative: ageing with intention

It's easy to brush off thoughts of ageing when we're in our 20s and 30s, when we're full of beans and often enjoying a clean bill of health. But the fact that you're here reading this suggests you're already invested in making choices that support your health and longevity.

If we approach ageing with doom and gloom, that's the energy we feed into our bodies. You are as young as you feel - so how old *do* you feel? Research on epigenetics now reinforces the fact that we have more control on how we age than we once thought. Our thoughts, relationships, habits and *milieu*, the social environment we immerse ourselves in, all shape the way our genes express over time. One of the most powerful things you can do is surround yourself with uplifting, like-minded people - those who see ageing as an opportunity for growth, not decline.

Pro-ageing exercise: reflect on your beliefs

By shedding light on our ageing beliefs, we can see what uplifts us and what holds us back. Take a moment to reflect here:

1. Without censoring or judgement, write down three beliefs you currently hold about ageing - just observe what comes up.
2. Now ask yourself: *Where did those beliefs come from?* Are they yours, or were they inherited from society, family or the media?
3. Choose one belief you'd like to reframe and write a new, empowering version of it.

Examples of ageing mindset reframing:

- *Ageing means slowing down* becomes *Ageing invites me to live with more depth and wisdom.*
- *I'm too old to start something new* becomes *I'm excited to explore new passions and opportunities.*
- *Ageing means becoming irrelevant* becomes *With age comes lived wisdom and I feel valued.*

Gratitude brings powerful transformation

In *Āyurveda*, *anukampā* - meaning compassion, grace and gratitude - is seen as an essential quality that softens the heart, sharpens the mind and uplifts the spirit. The beautiful thing is that gratitude is simple. It doesn't require a course or special tools, just a moment of presence. In many ways gratitude is the antithesis of fear-based ageing. And the more we practise it, the more it ripples outwardly. It's contagious.

Modern research echoes ancient wisdom traditions that people who regularly practise gratitude tend to sleep better, feel less anxious or low and even experience less physical pain. Something as simple as ending the day by noting three things you're grateful for can gently shift your entire outlook on life.

Of course, there will be days when gratitude feels out of reach. Days that are, frankly, just a bit shit. Those moments are part of life too. They're here to teach us resilience, to help us develop grit and cultivate hope and belief in better days ahead. It's OK to feel it all – the frustration, the sadness, the heaviness. Just don't get *stuck* there. Gratitude doesn't bypass pain, but it does help us move through it with a little more lightness.

When I think about my own ancestry, I'm in awe of the grit it must have taken to move across continents and start a new life with very little. I remind myself that this strength resides in me too. Sometimes we just need a moment to reflect. You're in the driver's seat of your journey and the practices in this book are designed to strengthen your inner grit and encourage both agency and a more positive outlook.

Pro-ageing exercise: daily gratitude

Each evening, write down three things you're grateful for, big or small. On tough days, start with something simple like your breath, a random encounter, a moment of silence. Over time, this practice gently rewires the brain to notice what's good, even when it feels like nothing is. Here are some prompts to get you started:

- *What am I most grateful for in my body today?*
- *What moment made me feel seen, safe or supported today?*
- *What challenge taught me something about myself recently?*
- *In what way did I connect with nature today?*
- *What ancestral quality or strength lives within me?*

Start small, keep it simple

If you're unsure how to start creating more stillness in your day, your mornings are a powerful place to begin. How you start your day shapes the energy you carry into the world. A few minutes of breathwork, a gratitude note or simple *dinacaryā* (daily) rituals can anchor you in presence.

Instead of reaching for your phone and inviting in the noise of the world before you're even out of bed, try pausing. Check in with yourself. Set a gentle intention such as: *I choose to be calm and focused today.* Breathe. Stretch. Sip your tea with awareness. Small actions, done with love, create a different kind of momentum.

Pillar 6

Sense and sensibility

'We may encounter many defeats, but we must not be defeated.'

Maya Angelou

We are each a complete ecosystem, interconnected, layered and ever-changing. So, when it comes to health, healing and ageing, our approach must be just as all-encompassing. *Āyurveda*'s definition of health (*see* pp. 37–8) is a powerful reminder of this. Alongside the expected physical and mental markers, it includes *prasanna ātmā indriya manaḥ,* which means a clear and contented soul, sharp and harmonious senses, and a peaceful mind (as mentioned in pillar 5). True well-being, in other words, touches every part of who we are.

In Pillar 6, we explore three often-overlooked components of lasting vitality. These elements might not show up in blood tests or be measured by fitness trackers, but they gradually impact how we age. They are:

- Sensory well-being – how to care for the senses through a mindful 'sensory diet' and nourishing rituals
- Emotional equanimity – why unprocessed emotions accelerate ageing and simple ways to cultivate calm and clarity for resilience
- Social nourishment – exploring the rejuvenating power of meaningful connection and relationships.

Each of these influences how *fully* we live, not just how long. Let's unfold them together.

Sensory well-being

The five senses are our portals of perception to the outside world. Caring for them both physically and filtering what we allow into our inner world are sure-found ways to preserve and protect vitality. Let's understand both aspects.

What's in your sensory diet?

In *Āyurveda*, digestion is not limited to food alone. It's also about what we ingest through our eyes, ears, nose, tongue and skin (known as our *jñānendriya)*, or organs of knowledge. Our five senses do more than passively receive external impressions: they are gatekeepers through which our mind, emotions and nervous system are shaped. Every part of us - our skin, heart, gut, even our hormonal system - is affected by the quality of sensory input. Through them, we experience the five subtle elements (*tanmātras*): sound, touch, form, taste and smell. Over time, these impressions shape how we feel in the moment and how we respond to life itself. In the context of *rasāyana*, nurturing our senses isn't a luxury, it's a cornerstone of disease-prevention and conscious ageing.

Sensory impressions move through the gross body (physical body) and our subtle body (mind and energy field) and must be processed, just like food. If left, they linger like *āma,* but as undigested impressions that cloud the mind, deplete energy and disturb our balance. In this way, your 'sensory diet' becomes just as vital to pro-ageing as what's on your plate.

As we mature, our faculties (*indriyas*) naturally begin to weaken. Classical texts describe *'asātmya-indriyārtha-saṃyoga',* which refers to the overuse, underuse or misuse of our senses as one of the key causes of imbalance and accelerated ageing. Overstimulation from digital excess or living in a cluttered environment can overload the system, leading to mental fog, emotional reactivity and fatigue (excess *rajas* or *tamas*). I like to think of sharp senses as well-tuned instruments, helping us stay in harmony with life's orchestra - provided we make wiser, more aligned choices. *See* Table 11.1 on pp. 216–17 for a breakdown of how our senses become imbalanced and ways to rebalance.

A filtered sensory diet helps preserve *ojas*, protect *prāṇa* and calm the mind by cultivating *sattva* (clarity) while minimising *rajas* (overstimulation) and *tamas* (dullness). When our senses are clear and well-nourished, we feel sharp, steady and connected – a powerful pro-ageing trio.

A healthy sensory diet means we are intentional about:

- What we listen to (music, conversation, silence)
- What we touch (textures, temperature, human connection)
- What we see (visual media, colours, nature's beauty)
- What we taste (flavours, food quality)
- What we smell (aromas, environments).

Each of our five senses corresponds to one of the five elements (*pañca mahābhūtas*): *ākāśa* (ether), *vayu* (air), *tejas* (fire), *jala* (water) and *pṛthvī* (earth). Let's consider each one more closely.

Sound (*ākāśa*/ether)

Perceived through the ears, sound is linked to ether, the subtlest element through which vibration travels. In everyday life, our ears constantly absorb unfiltered noise – news, traffic, notifications, chatter, that unconsciously dysregulate our nervous system. Unlike our eyes, which we can close to find relief, our ears remain open, making it harder to find stillness. That's why conscious listening practices like mantra, singing bowls or simply tuning into the breath can act as a filter and bring instant calm.

Touch (*vayu*/air)

Felt through the skin, touch is associated with air. As our largest and most sensitive organ, our skin is constantly communicating pressure, temperature, pain and many subtle sensations. A warm embrace, a gentle massage or a warm bath and feeling soft natural fabrics on the skin can all bring grounding and calm to the nervous system. In a world of growing digital dissonance, touch remains a powerful anchor for safety, belonging and comfort.

Did you know your skin makes up about 15 per cent of your total body weight?

Sight (*tejas*/fire)

Governed by the fire element, sight is our most dominant sense and often described as the windows to the soul. *Ācārya* Suśruta, known as the 'father of surgery', says that we absorb most of our outer world through the eyes. Today, however, our eyes are relentlessly overstimulated by artificial light from all angles, resulting in a severely scattered mind. Eye-care rituals like palming (eye relaxation technique), working with natural light, using rose water compresses or resting in darkness helps cool and soothe this fiery sense.

Taste (*jala*/water)

Experienced through our tongue, taste is linked to water and is essential for nourishment and digestion. Beyond identifying flavours, it activates digestion (via the gut–brain axis) and influences mood. Our palate today has become accustomed to excess, sugar, salt and spice, and perhaps we've forgotten what natural foods taste like. Mindful eating, savouring meals with all six tastes and avoiding rushed or emotion-driven snacking keeps this sense sharp and our digestive fire strong.

Did you know? Your tongue is a muscular organ, covered in thousands of taste buds – typically between 2000 and 8000.

Smell (*pṛthvī*/earth)

Received through the nose, smell is the earth element sense; it links directly to our brain and emotions, so the nasal passages act as a gateway for influencing the brain and senses. Whether through *prāṇāyāma* (breathwork and energy regulation), aromatherapy or simply inhaling the scent of fresh air, flowers or herbs, a single scent can calm the nerves, lift our mood or spark nostalgia.

Why sensory care matters

Our senses aren't meant to absorb everything; they're designed to filter only what truly serves us. This natural filtering protects us from sensory overload. Similar to how we hear only a slice of the sound spectrum or see only a narrow range of light (excluding UV or IR), our senses are our bodyguards, functioning best when we have awareness.

When our senses are neglected, strained or overstimulated, sharpness fades and imbalance begins. The key is to notice the early signs of sensory imbalance and gently guide them back to harmony. Use Table 11.1 below and overleaf as a quick guide to take better sensory care:

Sense	Causes of imbalance	Restorative practices
Sound *(śrotra)* Organ: Ears Element: Ether	Constant background noise or loud environments can cause irritation, anxiety or overwhelm. Energetically, sound imbalances mute inner listening and intuition.	Practise listening to nature's calming soundscape, mantras or soothing music. Perform *karṇa-pūraṇa* (oiling of the ears) with warm sesame or herbal oils. Explore sound healing.
Touch *(sparśa)* Organ: Skin Element: Air	Lack of a gentle, nurturing touch, harsh stimulation or stressful environments can leave us feeling restless or hypersensitive.	Regular *abhyanga* (self-massage) with warm oils tailored to your *doṣa*, wearing comfortable clothing and experiencing nature's textures (sand, breeze, sun, water, grass) help nurture this sense. Explore contact dance and soulful intimacy.
Sight *(cakṣus)* Organ: Eyes Element: Fire	Overexposure to bright lights, screens or visual stress can cause eye strain, dryness and poor vision. It may show up as confusion and dullness or lack of mental clarity.	Close your eyes and splash your face with cool water. Do cool rose water compresses, *nasya* (nasal oiling) to lubricate internally, or gentle eye exercises. Try warm oil foot massage at night to calm and nourish the eyes, and don't overlook the importance of good sleep.

→

Sense	Causes of imbalance	Restorative practices
Taste *(rasa)* Organ: Tongue Element: Water	Overindulgence or lack of variety in flavours can lead to digestive imbalance, cravings, aversions or emotional imbalance. It may inhibit our appetite for life.	Consume fresh, seasonal and wholesome foods that have a balance of all six tastes (sweet, sour, salty, pungent, bitter, astringent). Chew thoroughly and mindfully to savour each bite. *Āyurveda* advocates *jihvā-nirlekhana* (tongue scraping) and ***kavala*** (oil pulling) to clear *āma* and enliven taste buds. Explore mindful cooking.
Smell *(ghrāṇa)* Organ: Nose Element: Earth	Exposure to pollution or synthetic scents may dull the sense of smell, leading to respiratory or emotional discomfort. It may reduce our sense of feeling grounded and result in headaches.	Use natural fragrances such as essential oils, fresh flowers or herbal incense. Practise *jala neti* (nasal cleansing with salt water) and *nasya* (nasal oil therapy). Explore aromatherapy.

Table 11.1 Sensory balance and imbalance

By choosing simple and intentional sensory inputs, we restore balance. So, let's turn our attention now to how we can physically care for each of these vital gateways.

Morning rituals to awaken senses

These daily *Āyurvedic* morning cleansing rituals (*dinacharyā*) help to wake up your senses, through which you meet the world. If you have existing conditions affecting the ears, nose, mouth, skin or eyes, consult your practitioner for guidance.

Danta dhāvana (cleaning teeth)

We wouldn't start the day without brushing our teeth, but did you know that keeping the whole mouth clean also supports healthy digestion and immunity? Traditionally, fresh twigs of the neem tree were used to clean teeth and gums, a ritual considered to awaken taste perception.

How: Try an *Āyurvedic* herbal toothpaste or powder with ingredients that are naturally antibacterial, antiviral, antifungal and antimicrobial, such as neem, clove, liquorice, tulsi, triphala, cardamon, camphor or peppermint. Brush gently but thoroughly, floss daily and follow by tongue scraping and oil pulling (*see* below). You can also massage the gums with a drop of clove or neem oil for extra protection.

Jihvā-nirlekhana (tongue scraping)

Overnight, the tongue accumulates toxins (*āma*) that appear as a coating. Scraping the tongue first thing in the morning stimulates digestion, removes bacteria and awakens taste perception.

How: Use a stainless-steel or copper tongue scraper (*see* Resources). Gently scrape from the back to the front of the tongue five to seven times, rinsing between strokes.

Kavala (oil pulling)

This traditional mouth rinse helps remove toxins from the mouth, strengthens gums, lubricates the jaw and throat and enhances taste perception.

How: Take 1 tablespoon of warm cured sesame oil, *arimedādi taila* (*Āyurvedic* medicated oil) *or* coconut oil. Swish in the mouth for five to 10 minutes. Spit it out, then rinse the mouth with warm water (do not swallow the water).

Jala neti (nasal rinsing)

This saline rinse clears dust, pollen and congestion from the nasal passages, enhancing breathing, mental clarity and sharpening our sense of smell.

How: Use a ***neti* pot** with warm, sterile salt water (1 teaspoon of non-iodised [or sea/rock] salt per 500 ml of warm water). Tilt your head and pour gently through one nostril, allowing it to flow out the other, then repeat on the other side. Follow with *nasya* (*see* next page).

Nasya (nasal oiling)

Lubricating deep into the nasal passages supports mental clarity, lifts the mood, supports the nervous system and sharpens the sense of smell.

How: Lie back and place one to two drops of warm, medicated oil (such as *anu tailam* – *see* Resources) in each nostril. Inhale gently and deeply, then rest for a few minutes.

Netra prakṣālana (eye rinsing)

The eyes are the primary site of *pittā*, so cooling and cleansing them helps reduce strain, removes overnight accumulations in the corner of the eyes and overall, brightens the sense of sight.

How: Simply awaken by rinsing your whole face with cool water, with your eyes closed. Soothe the eyes with rose water compresses. *Nasya* (as above) also helps the eyes by supporting tear lubrication and relieving strain.

Karṇa-pūraṇa (ear oiling)

As we age, *vāta* tends to accumulate in the ears, leading to dryness, ringing or even anxiety. This practice grounds and soothes the nervous system and nourishes our sense of hearing.

How: Slightly warm some *cured* sesame oil.* Tilt your head and place two drops in one ear, then gently massage around the ear. Let it sit for a minute, then place cotton wool at the entrance to the ear canal and repeat on the other side. This is best done in the evenings, two to three times weekly. *Cured sesame oil (***mūrchita taila***) – a heat-processed oil in which impurities are removed, making it lighter, more stable and penetrative.

Udvartana and *abhyanga* (body scrub and massage)

Regular self-massage with warm herbal oils or powder cleanses and nourishes the skin, supports lymphatic flow and drainage, and restores radiance (*see* pp. 175–6 for a facial *ubṭana* recipe). This ritual strengthens immunity and nurtures the sense of touch.

How: Start with *udvartana*, a dry herbal massage using powders like *triphala*, turmeric, neem and sandalwood to exfoliate, stimulate circulation and reduce puffiness or stagnation. Or for convenience nowadays, use a dry body brush. Follow with an *abhyanga* – a nourishing warm oil massage.

Emotional equanimity

Just as our senses filter the world around us, our emotions filter our world within. So, let's now turn to our emotional diet: the subtle impressions that shape how we feel, heal, interact and age.

What's in your emotional diet?

Emotions are the language of the soul. Just as food nourishes the body, our emotions deeply influence our mental and spiritual well-being. It's helpful to remember that the word 'emotion' comes from the Latin '*e*' (out) and '*motion*' (move) – a reminder that emotions are meant to flow, not fester. Are you feeding your soul with joy and laughter, or are you weighed down by stress and negativity?

Life has a way of throwing many emotional curveballs our way: grief from a loss, the dread of loneliness, the heartache of a break-up, the anxiety of financial pressures or the disappointment of a missed opportunity. These moments are of course an inevitable part of our human journey and perhaps we're here to experience the full range of emotions. But the way we handle emotional unrest can either debilitate us or trigger growth. Imagine your emotional health as a garden. If we neglect it, the weeds can quickly spread, but as we tend to it with care, it can bud and bloom beautifully.

We often underestimate just how deeply our emotions impact us. Many of us were taught to value intellect over feelings, to think clearly but not necessarily to feel fully. As children, many of us were taught that emotions, especially those seen as negative, were not OK, being told 'don't cry', 'don't be sad/angry', 'don't be sensitive' or 'be brave'.

Emotional disturbances indirectly cause just as much suffering if not more than physical health. When we react emotionally, our responses are automatic and visceral, flooding the brain and body with chemical messengers linked to the stress response. They take over the rational mind and plug into something we can recall or relate to from our personal history, often learned in childhood. We continue to recreate history in our current situations, what is referred to as 'transference'.

When negative emotions are left unprocessed, they become lodged in the body. In *Āyurveda* these stored impressions are known as *saṃskāras*, the emotional imprints that discreetly shape our patterns, reactions and self-understanding over time (*see* pillar 7).

Stuck or unprocessed emotions can slowly (or quickly) manifest into physical health issues. Research shows clear links to digestive issues (IBS) and headaches. At a systemic level, chronic emotional stress can weaken immunity, impair digestion and accelerate ageing. Research on grief, for example, has been shown to depress immune function and increase susceptibility to illness.

Sadness often arises from regrets or loss. Anger shows up when our needs aren't met or we feel unseen. Fear and anxiety comes from feeling unprepared for what's ahead, or from perceived threats. These aren't weaknesses. Negative emotions are a natural part of being human. Just as we wisely choose food for physical health, we can also learn to recognise, feel and gently release disruptive emotional patterns to better support our inner well-being.

Slow down for what matters!

The first step in cultivating a healthier emotional diet is slowing down. In our rush to 'fix' things or distract ourselves from pain, we often overlook the value of simply being present with our feelings. When we pause long enough to notice them, emotions can become our deepest teachers. Grief reminds us of how deeply we love, anger signals a need to establish boundaries and fear encourages us towards breakthrough and growth. Noticing these messages is the first step; the next is learning how to bounce back and restore balance, what we call 'emotional resilience'.

Emotional resilience is not about avoiding pain or pushing through at all costs but moving through life's difficulties with awareness. Journalling, meditation, talking to a friend or seeking therapy are ways of metabolising experiences. Gratitude journalling in particular (as discussed in pillar 5) shifts our focus from what's wrong to being at peace with what is, creating space and allowing ourselves to feel joy again. Creativity, nature, human connection and rest are superfoods for our heart.

Emotional nourishment is not only processing the difficult feelings but also filling our cup with joy, laughter and lightness – vitamins for the soul. Laughter really is medicine, shown to lower stress hormones, boost immunity and even relieve pain. When was the last time you laughed so hard your belly ached? If it's been a while, maybe it's time to give yourself permission to feel it again. Watch a silly movie, play with your kids, or reminisce about funny memories with friends.

Even something as simple as a smile can work wonders. A smile, real or forced, sends signals to your brain to feel happier. Smiling more often can reduce stress, lower blood pressure and lift your spirits. Try smiling at a stranger on the street, yourself in the mirror or that bird outside your window.

Ultimately, slowing down helps us check in with what's on our emotional plate. Is it joy, stress or a little of both? And is your emotional diet truly nourishing your soul?

The power of dreams

Dreaming is one of the ways our mind processes and releases hidden or unexpressed emotions, gently sorting through experiences that we might not fully process while we're awake. During REM sleep, usually between 2 and 6 a.m., the mind's creative and healing pathways are most active, helping us to restore balance. Have you noticed what comes up in your dreams?

Pro-ageing exercise: cultivating inner strength

Take a quiet moment to notice an emotion that you are currently experiencing. Pause with it. It may be grief, anger or fear. Whatever arises, simply allow yourself to sit with it and feel it fully. Can you accept and allow it to be, without needing to change it?

Now see if you can experience that emotion as a vibration moving through you, rather than something you are. Feel into the space between who you are and what you are experiencing. In that space lies the invitation to respond differently and not just by default. This is the essence of detachment - where you are able to witness emotions with compassion and to recognise their impermanence - *anitya*.

Sometimes emotions get stuck in the body, so it can help to give the body a voice - a chance to express what the mind struggles to. The practices that follow are simple ways to open that flow.

Pro-ageing exercise: dynamic movement for release

Here is a simple somatic movement technique to help you release stuck energy from the nervous system, especially if you have negative emotions. This practice helps discharge the stress response and re-ground the body - great at the end of a tough day or after conflict.

1. Put on energising or cathartic music if you wish.
2. Stand with your feet hip-width apart. Close your eyes if it feels comfortable.
3. Begin to gently bounce or shake your body, starting from your knees and letting the movement travel upwards. If it feels right, let your arms move freely, let them rise, dangle and shake. Keep your jaw relaxed and shoulders loose.
4. Breathe naturally or exhale audibly through your mouth.

→

5. After two to three minutes, slow down gradually. Pause, place a hand on your heart or belly or both, and notice how you feel. Allow your negative emotions to float away. You may wish to say a comforting affirmation or lie down.
6. Gently bring your awareness back into the room and open your eyes.

Pro-ageing exercise: *Siṁha Prāṇāyāma* – lion's breath and vocal release

This breath-based technique taps into the vagus nerve and helps release emotional tension stored in the chest, jaw and diaphragm:

1. Kneel comfortably in *Siṁhāsana* (Lion Pose).
2. Inhale deeply through the nose.
3. As you exhale, open your mouth wide, stick out your tongue and let out a long, strong and loud *haaah* sound, like a sigh from deep in your belly. Let your face, jaw and chest soften as you retract.
4. Repeat four or five times, then pause and notice how you feel.

Social nourishment

Just as our emotions need space and nourishment, so too does our need for connection. We aren't meant to walk through life alone, so let's explore the role of community and meaningful relationships in supporting pro-ageing. The more conscious we become of our social inputs, the more we can lean into relationships that uplift us, create boundaries around those who drain us and open space for new connections that truly nourish. So, let's first take a moment to notice your social patterns.

Pro-ageing exercise: curating your social diet

To help you nurture a social diet that feels nourishing, connected and inspired, ask yourself the following questions:

1. Who do I spend the most time with each week?
2. Which of these relationships feels energising or joyful and which feels draining?
3. What kind of support or connection am I needing more of?
4. How can I create space for meaningful connection (or solitude) in the week ahead?
5. Is there a community group or act of service I feel drawn to explore?

What's in your social diet?

As humans, we are inherently social beings. Throughout life, we play many roles - the child, sibling, friend, parent, partner, colleague, neighbour - and each one adding to our sense of belonging. The people we surround ourselves with will influence our daily lives and our long-term well-being.

Our social 'diet' is made up of the relationships and interactions we feed on daily and it nourishes us as much as our physical, mental and emotional diet. It includes family, friends, work colleagues, community, spiritual groups, and yes, even the time we spend with ourselves. It also includes our digital connections, which these days are expanding faster than our real-life ones. Although they offer convenience and reach, virtual connections often come at the cost of depth and presence.

A truly nourishing social diet supports our emotional resilience, which we discussed earlier on pp. 221–222, cognitive health, which we explored in pillar 5, and vitality as we age. But like all forms of nourishment, it requires awareness and intention.

Community and connection for pro-ageing

If you asked me what caused the greatest harm to our collective well-being during the pandemic, I'd say it wasn't just the virus or the fear but the breakdown of community, connection and joy.

Connection is not just a 'nice-to-have' – it's vital. *Āyurveda*, along with other ancient traditions, reminds us that healing doesn't happen in isolation. We thrive when we feel seen, heard and supported. In Sanskrit, the word ***satsaṅga*** refers to a gathering of truth, where a community of like-minded individuals come together to share wisdom and nurture meaningful relationships. Whether through spiritual circles or shared meals, *satsaṅga* sustains positivity, inspiration and emotional resilience, creating an environment where both personal growth and communal harmony flourishes. In fact, nearly all respondents in my over-60s survey emphasise the importance of relationships, family and community for health and fulfilment.

We're wired for connection and the Social Baseline Theory, which suggests that humans are biologically built to conserve energy and feel safer through social bonds, recognises it as part of our human design. Staying connected helps you adapt, stay grounded and handle life's ups and downs with more ease. Many respondents from my research rate relationships as 'very important' or 'integral' to their quality of life and several note that volunteering or community involvement has become more meaningful with age. However, some acknowledge that opportunities for new social connection can diminish with age and there is concern about societal undervaluing of elders.

Society plays a powerful role in shaping how we perceive ageing, especially through media and cultural norms. Respondents highlighted negative framing of women's ageing, with one noting, 'society is hugely influential in how we view female ageing'. At the same time, family, friends, books and trusted online voices were often considered as positive influences.

You become who you spend time with, so it's worth asking: *Who am I regularly in contact with? Do these connections uplift, inspire and reflect the person I'm becoming? Or am I hanging on to relationships purely out of familiarity, even when they've become relics of a past version of myself?*

Community as a healing ecosystem

Let's unpack some simple yet powerful ways to forge meaningful connections in your daily life. This might be through:

- **Sitting in a circle of wisdom** with others, young and old, sharing stories, listening deeply and learning from each other's journeys.
- **Honouring life transitions with rituals** (like the traditional rites of passage – birth, coming of age, marriage, parenthood or stepping into wisdomhood). These collective moments open space to recognise and celebrate life's chapters with loved ones.
- **Volunteering your time** to something that matters. Whether planting in a community garden or serving a warm meal at a soup kitchen, it helps us to feel that we belong, and that our contribution counts.
- **Sharing joy together** by moving together, singing, dancing or laughing around a table (*satsaṅga*). These small, joyful moments reconnect us to each other while soothing our nervous system.
- **Creating new connections** through activities that align with your passions, such as yoga, book clubs, festivals or cultural groups (*see* pillar 5 for more).
- **Small, thoughtful gestures**, such as checking in on a neighbour or sharing a simple cup of tea with a friend in need can be deeply nourishing.

Whether it's engaging in ritual, laughter, service or small everyday gestures, it's the awakened sense of belonging that matters most. We thrive when we have the right meaningful social connections. When balanced with space for reflection, rest and self-love rituals, we create the perfect recipe for our emotional, mental and physical well-being.

Honouring wisdomhood (*sannyāsa*)

At my half-centenarian stage in life, I've noticed how different our relationship with our elders looks now compared to when I was growing up. Census data show that in 2021 around 279,000 people aged 65-plus lived in care homes in England and Wales, rising to over 350,000 residents in care homes across England by mid-2025. This reality is such a contrast to one of my most treasured memories from my childhood – seeing how our elders were cherished at the centre of family life. They were cared for by their children and grandchildren and were respected as wisdom-keepers.

This sense of family and community spirit still exists in many cultures around the world today, but as we become 'busier' in life and health challenges increase, the model of care homes is becoming more prevalent and normalised. In contrast, many eastern traditions honour ageing not as a decline or burden, but as a form of 'life promotion'. Elders impart knowledge, guide and support families and community as they embrace their *sannyāsa* stage of life.

Pillar 7

Soul-nourishing secrets

'The spirit within us is the only all-efficient doctor and submission of the body to it the one true panacea.'

Sri Aurobindo

Ageing as a spiritual journey

Buddha said that life is full of suffering, but are we really doomed from womb to tomb? If we continue to live in a state of 'life happens to me' then perhaps this statement will feel true. But he also expressed that it is possible to overcome suffering by self-awareness and spiritual evolution, and this is exactly the premise of the pro-ageing growth journey and the focus of this pillar.

The previous pillars focused on the more tangible 'doing' aspects of caring for your mind, body and senses to close in on the 'vitality gap'. *Rasāyana*, however, is not limited to food, herbs and longevity rituals. Its deepest power lies in the intangible nectar that nourishes the soul, what we call *adhyātmika*. Through pillar 7, we explore how ageing, when embraced as a spiritual journey, becomes the ultimate *rasāyana*, turning life itself into medicine that's deeply transformative. It is made of practices of 'being' that are often overlooked in the modern wellness world but safeguard against despair, disconnection and fear – factors that no prescription can remedy. At the same time, they instil hope, faith and enthusiasm for life. Here we enter the realm of the inner *kośas* (*see* pp. 67–70), exploring soul-nourishing *rasāyana* practices such as purpose, forgiveness, play, faith, detachment and conscious preparation for death. Together they prepare us to both live well and age with grace.

In this pillar we will understand:

- The power of realising your *dharma* and living in alignment with your deeper purpose
- Moving from labels to liberation through the art of letting go, embracing impermanence and embodying kindness
- Anchoring into the unseen through faith, prayer and rituals for inner peace
- Emotional composting – clearing *karma* and transforming *saṃskāra*
- The fortunes of forgiveness to release what no longer serves
- Living with ***līlā*** to cultivate joy, play and childlike wonder
- The art of dying well – preparing for spiritual liberation.

Some people seem to radiate a deep joy and presence, making you think, *they've really got soul*. That same aliveness is available to us all when we begin to open to a more expansive view of life.

Ageing is not just physical process but a profound invitation to release, awaken and deepen, spiritually. Working on this pillar presents you with an opportunity to continually ask yourself the bigger questions: *Who am I beyond my roles? What truly matters? How do I prepare for what comes next, both externally and internally? What is the purpose of my existence? What do I desire? What drives me? What sparks joy? What stimulates the 'feel-good' factor beyond my material desires? What holds me back? And what heals me at a deeper level? And ultimately, what fuels my journey and brings peace to my soul?*

Through the Vedic lens, ageing is not a decline but a ripening of our soul and preparation for the sacred art of dying well (*antim sañskāra*). This inner work is vital to pro-ageing. For me at least, *this* is the journey of well-being, and in the following pages, I invite you to deeply explore profound Vedic wisdom and soulful practices that support your personal growth.

The power of realising your *dharma*

In chapter 4, I proposed that you set a *saṅkalpa*, your sacred vow. Now let's return to that inner commitment that is deeply connected to *dharma* as we ask: *What am I really here to express in this life? What gives my days meaning?* While realising our purpose can't be rushed or forced, it does become clearer the more we listen, reflect and live with intention.

Just as the bees and trees have their unique nature and purpose, so too do you! The *dharma* of bees is to pollinate plants, facilitating their reproduction and contributing to the ecosystem balance. Trees produce oxygen, absorb carbon dioxide and provide shade and habitat for numerous species. Your *dharma* (accurately: *svadharma*) is to discover, nurture and share your natural gifts. It's a way of aligning your life with the greater order of the universe, an idea rooted in the *Ṛgveda*, one of the oldest Vedic texts. And when you do, life often feels more at ease.

Your *dharma* isn't limited to a job title or identity. It's deeper than that. It's the sacred call of your soul, the path that aligns with who you truly are beneath your roles and responsibilities. You might express it through work, creativity or service, but the essence remains the same: it's living in tune with your true nature and the flow of life.

At its highest level, *dharma* becomes a spiritual path. It's a shift from acting out of habit or fear to navigating from awareness and clarity. The ego makes space for something more timeless to take the lead: our consciousness.

Living by our own inner compass rather than cultural doctrines or collective pressures is how we begin to claim spiritual sovereignty. *Dharma* becomes a guide not just for what we do, but how we live, love and discern.

In early life, *dharma* often centres around your personal growth and contribution to family, society and the world. But as the years pass, the focus naturally expands. *Dharma* becomes more universal, centred on service, spiritual evolution and connection to the greater whole.

Dharma is essentially the 'right' way to live, a way of aligning with your highest purpose to ensure stability in your external environment. While *dharma* might seem predetermined, strong intuition and free will can help you discover and redirect your life purpose, allowing you to experience effortless flow.

As we learned in chapter 4, each life stage (*āśramas*) carries its own *dharma*: learning and discipline in youth (*brahmacharya*); responsibility and service in midlife (*gṛhastha*); reflection and spiritual focus in later years (*vānaprastha*); and ultimately, wisdom and self-realisation in the mature years (*sannyāsa*). Each phase supports the soul's evolution towards inner freedom.

Pro-aging exercise: Finding your true path

Living in alignment with your *dharma* strengthens your vitality (*ojas*, *tejas* and *prāṇa*). Ideally it arises from within, but this four-step exercise can support you through your discovery process. You can return to it any time.

1. When do you feel most alive and aligned? Think of those moments when time just flies by and what you're doing feels both joyful and meaningful. What experiences do you keep being drawn to?
2. What comes most naturally to you – the qualities, strengths, skills or knowledge that seem effortless and that others value in you?
3. Which *doṣa* reflects your nature?
   - *Vāta*: Creative, intuitive, expressive. You serve through vision and communication.
   - *Pittā*: Focused, determined, dynamic. You serve through leadership and problem-solving.
   - *Kapha*: Patient, nurturing, diligent. You serve through compassion, reliability and healing.
4. Complete the sentence: *'I bring more ___ into the world by ___.'*

Moving from labels to liberation: the art of letting go

Do you believe you are an eternal soul? Even if that idea feels far-fetched, consider for a moment – what if you are a soul having a human experience?

Vedic wisdom expresses, *'Aham Brahmasmi'* or 'I am Brahman' – the idea that I am a part of the infinite existence. Our name, job or status may offer a sense of security and belonging, but they can get in the way of knowing our deeper selves.

Everything is energy: becoming, transforming and dissolving. We are energetic beings vibrating at various frequencies. Yet, we become easily attached to our familiar material reality – our possessions, routines, desires, cravings, thoughts, emotions, past experiences and desired future.

These attachments can weigh us down and become the very source of our suffering. But what happens if we loosen our grip on them?

The Vedic truth of *anitya,* meaning impermanence, teaches us that everything is constantly changing, both in the world around us and in who we are becoming. We catch glimpses of this in fleeting moments of resonance – when you feel a spark with another person, only to watch it pass. Yet most of us will resist this reality. We cling to our roles and labels and wear them as badges of identity.

When we begin to accept impermanence, something shifts. We instantly become less reactive and feel lighter. There is space to breathe, to feel, to simply be. This is *vairāgya* (non-attachment). It is the release of the tight grip we have on our need for validation, expectations and control. When we lean into impermanence, letting go can feel more like an opening of inner peace than a loss. When we are no longer clinging, competing or comparing, acceptance and kindness become our most natural state.

Kindness as a spiritual currency

Kindness is contagious! Small acts of kindness create profound ripple effects. *Seva* (selfless service) embodies the spirit of altruism and a true sense of compassion towards others. Being a humble human is at the root of *seva* and is considered a vital aspect of our spiritual development. True *seva* is an attitude of being of service without any need for recognition or a sense accomplishment; it is completely selfless and an integral part of *Sadvṛtta* (ethical and lifestyle conduct) in the *Caraka Saṃhitā* that is said to lead to longevity, strength (*bala*) and happiness (*sukha*). *Seva* is the ultimate way to tame the ego and extend humility. Kindness isn't just good for others, it's a potent elixir to open our own heart. Data from the Wisconsin Longitudinal Study (1957–present), showed a 1.8% mortality rate among altruistic volunteers compared to 4.3% among non-volunteers, demonstrating that genuine concern for others substantially reduces mortality risk.

It releases oxytocin and reduces blood pressure, cortisol and inflammation, protecting us against chronic diseases and promoting longevity. Ask yourself how you can build a culture of *Seva* (selfless service) in your community.

Shraddhā and devotion: anchoring in the unseen

Shraddhā is the Sanskrit word often translated as faith, devotion and reverence that comes from deep within us. *Shrad* means 'truth' or 'faithfulness' and *dhā* means to 'hold' or 'support'. At its essence, *shraddhā* is the pathway that connects us with our higher self.

For much of my life, I understood *shraddhā* as faith in something outside of myself. Traditionally, it is expressed as an outward devotion to a god/goddess/deity, guided by religious institutions. But the nature of *shraddhā* runs much deeper for me. Today, I experience *shraddhā* as a deep inner devotion – the foundation of trust that compels me to act and guides my growth even when I cannot see the path ahead. For me now, it's less about faith in something external and more about faith in my higher self and in life's unfolding. Having said that, I am forever drawn to sacredness of rituals.

While *dharma* is the path we walk, *shraddhā* is the light that illuminates each step even when the full path isn't always clear. *Shraddhā* is the faith that keeps our inner and outer worlds aligned, allowing truth, emotion and purpose to flow as one.

In the context of pro-ageing, *shraddhā* becomes a subtle form of *rasāyana* and helps us soften our resistance and expand by 'trusting the process', surrendering to time and embracing the invisible intelligence of life. Take a moment to contemplate what *shraddhā* means for you and how it guides your choices, decisions and actions.

The power of prayer and rituals for inner peace

Prayer and ritual can be beautiful anchors for peace, clarity and connection. Whether you whisper prayers quietly to yourself or share rituals in a communal sacred space – I like to think of it as our 'faith flex'. Our mental and spiritual state shapes how we age and how we move through life's transitions. Practices like *japa* (mantra repetition), *bhakti* (devotion) and simple *smṛti* (mindfulness) can bring a deep sense of harmony, helping us to release our fears and loosen attachments. *Upāsana*, prayer or worship in any form, creates space for us to reconnect with something greater, whatever that may be for you.

It's not about following a fixed doctrine but about finding what feels sincere and nourishing. Light a candle, chant a word that opens your heart, offer flowers back to the earth or simply sit in stillness. These small rituals draw us into presence, deepening the connection to our soul – through *shraddhā*. When we pray together with shared intention, the connection strengthens, energy rises, consciousness is elevated and greater healing unfurls.

Clearing *karma* and the impact of *saṃskāras*

What drives us forwards in life? For some, it is *shraddhā* (faith) and *bhakti* (devotion), the invisible anchors that help us navigate uncertainty. For others, it's *dharma* that brings a sense of duty, purpose and moral compass. If we wish to move forward with clear direction and inner power, we must also tend to the hidden imprints that influence our course.

These karmic imprints are subtle impressions left behind from past actions, words, thoughts or emotions – much like footprints in wet sand. When we repeat the same actions, the impressions deepen and become embedded in the unconscious mind (*chitta*). Over time they become a pattern and subsequently become our conditioning called *saṃskāras*. These *saṃskāras* influence how we think, feel and act – think of it as our default learned behaviour. The Sanskrit roots of the words are *sam* (to 'come together') and *kār* ('action undertaken'), suggesting an accumulation of repeated experience.

Many *saṃskāras* are formed in our early childhood, even as early as the womb. *Saṃskāras* can be positive, carrying imprints of love, encouragement and belonging. These positive impressions create patterns of self-trust, kindness and confidence that help us flourish.

Other *saṃskāras* can be negative or harmful and are often the roots of our self-sabotaging patterns that can diminish self-worth, erode confidence, strain relationships and ultimately hold us back in life. In the *Yoga Sutra* (2:16), *Ācārya* Patañjali notes: *'Heyam duhkham anagatam'* – 'future suffering can be avoided'. Today, this highlights the importance of self-awareness and 'doing the inner work' to dissolve those deep-rooted patterns that we've come to accept as our emotional and behavioural default, but it's an invitation to break the cycle.

When these *saṃskāras* are left unresolved, they cloud our perception, robbing us of peace and vitality. By dissolving them with awareness, we make space for growth, conscious ageing and the possibility of rewriting our story with intention (*saṅkalpa*).

Round and round it goes in a looping pattern, from *saṃskāra* to ***vāsanā*** to *karma* and back to *saṃskāra,* as in Figure 12.1 below. This cycle continues until we interrupt the pattern with awareness and break the cycle. Let's take a moment to explore your own patterns and conditioning.

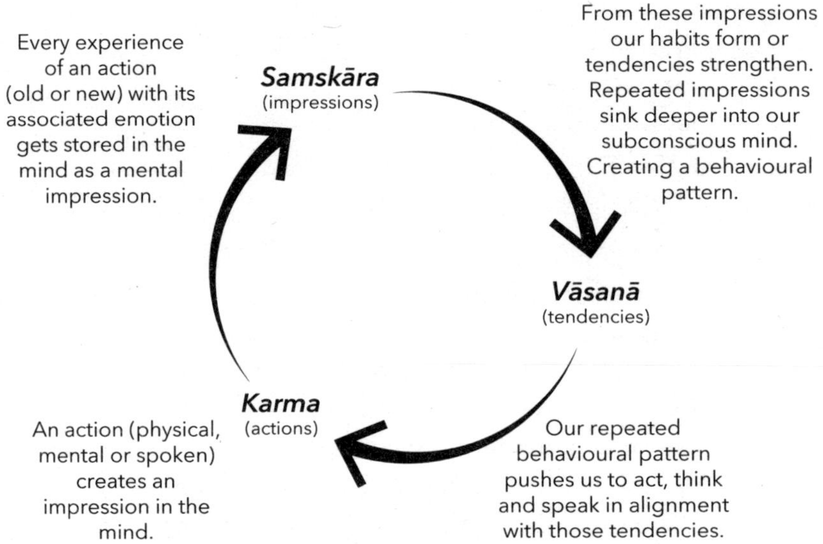
Every experience of an action (old or new) with its associated emotion gets stored in the mind as a mental impression.
Samskāra
(impressions)
From these impressions our habits form or tendencies strengthen. Repeated impressions sink deeper into our subconscious mind. Creating a behavioural pattern.
Vāsanā
(tendencies)
Karma
(actions)
An action (physical, mental or spoken) creates an impression in the mind.
Our repeated behavioural pattern pushes us to act, think and speak in alignment with those tendencies.

Figure 12.1 The cycle of *saṃskāra*, *vāsanā* and *karma*

Pro-ageing exercise: exploring your inner patterns

This self-inquiry exercise is designed to help you notice your *saṃskāras* and patterns (especially the negative ones) that may be shaping your default reactions, relationships or self-perception. The aim here is not to fix or analyse, but simply to *observe* with honesty and compassion.

You may then wish to use these as journalling prompts or bring them into a therapeutic or healing space. Whatever arises, let it come up without judgement.

Tips for reflection:

- There's no right answer, just curiosity.
- If a question stirs something, pause and stay with it.
- Consider noting down insights, sensations or memories that arise.

The prompts:

1. Do you often overlook your own achievements and rarely celebrate your wins?
2. Are there important relationships (with family, friends, partners or yourself) that feel fragile or unresolved?
3. Do you sometimes feel emotionally overwhelmed, or disconnected from your feelings?
4. How easily and how often do you feel angry, irritable or frustrated? Do you tend to express it outwardly (e.g. shouting), inwardly (e.g. self-criticism), or do you suppress it altogether?
5. Is it hard for you to share what you really feel, even with people close to you?
6. Do you ever feel a lack of love, support or true connection in your life?
7. Are you concerned about the future or possible changes?
8. Do you struggle to spend time in silence or alone, reaching for distractions to fill the void?
9. Do you find it difficult to let go of fears or move on from painful memories?
10. When you're feeling sad or down, do you tend to keep it in, feel and express it or supress it?

How to transform *saṃskāras*

Transformation begins with noticing your patterns, the stories you tell yourself, the triggers and the emotional hamster wheel you are stuck on. When you become aware of it, you can begin to release and heal. In the next section, we'll explore how forgiveness can melt away what's been held on to for too long and create space for something new to manifest.

Our strongest attractions or aversions – what we cling to or reject – often reveal *saṃskāras* at play. These aren't easily cleared simply by willpower or moral discipline. To truly release them, we must meet them where they live: in the subtle layers of our mind-body system.

Practices like meditation help us move beyond the surface, past thoughts and emotions into the deeper parts of our consciousness. This is where *saṃskāras* live. We might associate this with 'inner child healing' and 'shadow work'.

Imagine a child who grew up always being told they were never good enough, despite their efforts. Over time, this forms a *saṃskāra*: a belief that they are inadequate and is reflected in their behaviour. As an adult, this can show up as self-doubt, fear of failure or chronic people-pleasing.

Healing that *saṃskāra* begins with noticing the pattern and understanding where it comes from and offering compassion to the part of us that was hurt. The start of this journey might look like taking a walk with no prescribed destination, just following what feels right, or simply saying, *I am enough*. It's not about rejecting the past but about slowly dissolving its hold. For me, this work feels like a deep cleansing of emotional debris from the unconscious mind and it's an integral component of my well-being coaching with clients.

Modern modalities like self-hypnosis, trauma-informed therapy or somatic breathwork can also bring *saṃskāras* to the surface. When we observe what was once buried, with support, safety and awareness, only then can we rewire it.

Meditation practices like *Vipassanā* allow us to witness the *saṃskāra* as physical sensations, tightness, numbness, heat or even visions. When we stay with the sensation, without reacting or labelling, it begins to dissolve. What once felt stagnant becomes fluid and impermanent. Sometimes this awareness arises spontaneously in our day-to-day lives. A familiar reaction, a sudden fear, a moment of shutdown can all be clues. This becomes a pathway for us to shift our *karma* (actions) and reshape our *vāsanās* (tendencies).

The recent surge in access to psychedelic plant medicine, such as ayahuasca, huachuma (San Pedro) and peyote, can be powerful vehicles to access these hidden spaces of our mind and heart for deep inner work and healing, when held in a sacred and guided setting. Used with intention, these practices are worlds apart from the fleeting highs of recreational substances designed for escapism.

If you have reached a point in your therapy journey but sense there is deeper 'work' to do, then the practices of Indigenous healing traditions may be the path not yet explored. Many of these, including those rooted in the Vedas, use the elements of nature (space, air, water, fire, earth) to work at the level of the energy body (inner *kośas*), cleansing our mind-body, dissolving emotional imprints and releasing *saṃskāras*. Rituals can include fire offerings (*homa* or *agnihotra)*, water purification rites (*melukat* ceremonies), river immersions (*snāna*), mantra chanting (*nāda*), earth-based therapies (e.g. grounding), sweat lodges (*temazcal*) and smoke ceremonies (smudging) with herbs such as sage or copal. Over the years, I've felt profound stillness and release after a *homa*, a *melukat* in Bali and daily bathing in the river Gangā, along with other traditional energy-based practices.

When we do this inner work of clearing *samskāras*, we loosen old emotional debris, release what holds us down and can rewrite survival-driven patterns. This subsequently opens the door to mental clarity and graceful ageing, reflected in stronger immunity, reduced inflammation and cognitive resilience. When negative energy is dispelled, vitality naturally returns.

Supportive practices to deepen the journey

These additional tools that can be woven throughout the processes in this pillar to support and sustain your transformation:

Bhakti (devotion and surrender)

Lighten your inner work through love, prayer (*see* pp. 234–5), and mantras (*see* pp. 197–9). When willpower or awareness isn't enough, sometimes *saṃskāras* can be dissolved through love and devotion (*see* pp. 235–40).

Ancestral/intergeneration healing

Some *saṃskāras* aren't always yours, sometimes they could be inherited through karmic family patterns and collective traumas (intergenerational trauma). Rituals, forgiveness practices (*see* pp. 240–1) or prayer for one's lineage can help release inherited imprints by transforming how the past continues to impact our lives today.

→

Satsaṅga (conscious community)

Healing doesn't have to feel lonely. Being supported by a conscious community can help you stay steady and connected and acts as a mirror when old patterns resurface (*see* pp. 226–7). It can also be useful to have a small network of people who are supporting your journey. Most of all, though, be gentle and kind with yourself.

The fortune of forgiveness

It's inevitable that, over the course of our lives, we accumulate unresolved emotional baggage. Holding on to negative emotions such as anger, grief, sadness, resentment etc. can become the very poison that accelerates ageing, triggers disease and prevents healing or liberation. Why do we do it? Familiarity! One of the most profound tools for mental and emotional well-being is forgiveness. Forgiveness is not about excusing the harm caused but freeing yourself from the burden of carrying the often-destructive emotional weight. Supporting my clients through this process has truly paid dividends in how they feel, physically, mentally and emotionally. *Āyurveda* and modern research both highlight how unresolved emotions create stress, inflammation and premature ageing - remember the *pañca kośas* model in Figure 4.3 on p. 68? We are multidimensional beings with so many layers - each positively or negatively impacting the other. Bear this in mind as you use the prompts that follow to guide your inner work of release, renewal and self-compassion.

Pro-ageing exercise: discover what you're holding on to that no longer serves you

1. List any pain, anger, grudges or unresolved emotions you are still carrying from the past.
   - Observe how these feelings are showing up in your body - such as muscle tightness, palpitations, nausea, yawning, knot in the gut or sleep disturbances.

→

- Imagine lugging these feelings uphill in a heavy backpack. Now visualise taking off that backpack you've been hauling. What would life feel like without this bag?

2. What lesson can I take from this pain?
    - Reflect on whether this experience taught you something about self-worth, boundaries, guilt, blame or shame?
    - How can you transform these wounds into wisdom?
3. Who do I need to forgive (including myself) to move forwards?
    - Write a letter of self-forgiveness to yourself: 'I forgive myself for . . . I release myself from . . . I no longer allow . . .'. Keep going until you feel fully expressed.
4. How would my life change if I fully let go of this pain?
5. How would you feel physically, emotionally and mentally without these wounds weighing you down?

Living with *līlā* – the art of joy, play and childlike wonder

Youthfulness starts with play. When I observe the carefree attitude, innocence and freedom of children, I can't help but wonder if they truly hold the secrets to everlasting youth. As adults, play is often our lowest priority. Our lives are structured by endless 'to-do' lists rather than experiences of being. Play is both energy-raising and profoundly soul-stimulating. So how can we incorporate more play into our daily lives?

The Vedic idea of *līlā* refers to divine play. By embracing spontaneity, creativity and playfulness we have the ingredients to transform the mundane into magic and every moment shimmers with wonder and awe. *Līlā* has no set purpose, it's just the soul's expression of pure joy. Cultivating childlike wonder as a part of everyday spiritual practice, finding joy in new experiences and meeting life with curiosity, humour and light-heartedness is the most underrated mindset for pro-ageing.

In the *Bhagavad Gītā* and other Vedic texts, life is often described as a blend of purpose and *līlā*. As we follow our *dharma*, it's worth noting that the universe also moves with playfulness and to not take life too seriously. When we embrace both life's challenges and joys with the same light-hearted spirit, *līlā*, all experiences even the hardships are turned into part of a beautiful dance.

At its heart, *līlā* calls us to view life as a stage where each of us plays a part. While we may carry out our duties with devotion and focus, remember there's freedom beyond the duty and drama.

The Upanishads teaches us that the divine is both the creator and the observer of this cosmic play, helping us let go of ego-attachments and surrender to the flow of life – much like a dancer who loses herself in each step but remains rooted in the music.

Living with *līlā* encourages us to cultivate a playful energy in our day-to-day activities. Whether you are working, socialising or simply being, there's always room for spontaneity, creativity and joy, something guruji Sri Sri Ravi Shankar embodies so gracefully. Can you surrender to the play of life, trusting that every moment – whether joyful or challenging – is part of your soul's journey? Can you willingly embrace all of it?

Pro-ageing exercise: lighten up

Our days can become heavy and monotonous so reflect on where you might have become rigid in your outlook. Ask yourself where you can allow more playfulness and lightness into your life. Consider one small way you can introduce spontaneity today, for example:

- Put on a favourite song and dance for a few minutes.
- Call or message someone you haven't spoken to in a while.
- Buy some new fresh ingredients and experiment with a different dish.
- Take a walk or drive to somewhere new and people watch in a café.
- Put on that special outfit that never makes it out of your wardrobe – what are you saving it for?

The art of dying well: spiritual liberation

Death is an eventuality that is guaranteed for all of us and inseparable from the conversation of ageing as a spiritual journey. Yet it remains a subject that few want to discuss. Why is there such a taboo around death? Perhaps it is not death itself that we fear, but the *suffering* we may experience in the 'vitality gap'.

In *Āyurveda* and Vedic traditions, death is seen not as an end but a transition – a doorway to another cycle of existence – ***saṃsāra***. It is here that ageing well and dying well meet. The art of dying well is the culmination of intangible *rasāyana*, the final act of release, surrender and preparing for *mokṣa,* our ultimate freedom.

As Anita Moorjani articulates in her book *Dying to Be Me* about her personal near-death experience, death is not the end: we are an infinite existence, beyond our physical bodies. It's a beautiful transition indeed and accepting that is nothing short of an experience of pure unconditional love.

The process of conscious dying is deeply connected to how we live, age and prepare for ultimate liberation (*mokṣa*). Longevity (ā*yu*) in *Āyurveda* is not merely about extending life but about living meaningfully (including working through the ideas highlighted in this pillar) so that when our time comes, we can transition with grace, awareness and peace. Fear diminishes life. Love expands it.

Anita explains that her extraordinary recovery from end-stage cancer came from the realisation that her body had been absorbing years of fear, stress and self-rejection. The moment she let go of fear and aligned with love, her healing dramatically accelerated. She continues to encourage people to live fully *now*, rather than postponing joy for 'later' or living cautiously out of fear of dying, a pattern sometimes called 'deferred happiness syndrome'. What's interesting is that there is a universal acceptance across all cultures to offer the body back to the earth through fire, burial or other rites.

The *Bhagavad Gītā* (2.27) states that: 'For one who is born, death is certain; and for one who dies, birth is certain. Therefore, you should not grieve over the inevitable.'

With *shraddhā* (faith) and *bhakti* (devotion) as inner comrades, *saṅkalpa* as our guiding star and *dharma* as our conscious path, we can begin to reshape our inner landscape with *rasāyana*. Simultaneously, forgiveness softens our heart, *līlā* (playfulness) lightens our journey, *vairāgya* (detachment) frees us from clinging to temporary pleasures, while prayer keeps us anchored. Together, these teachings create the opportunity to embrace new patterns at every layer of our being, where ageing becomes a conscious choice and life is experienced as a celebration.

'You only live once, but if you work it right, once is enough.'
Joe E. Lewis

Final thoughts: celebrate you!

Ancient Indian philosophy holds that birthdays mark our entry into existence in our current human form, as well as another solar return. Whether you go with this or not, a birthday means one more year of wisdom! We may complain – 'Oh, another year older' or 'I'm getting old now' – but the reality is, we should be another year wiser. It's a great opportunity to reflect on our personal growth and development, not just review work, finances and outward accomplishments. Are we happier and healthier than the year before?

Rather than clinging to the past or resisting the inevitable, what if we embraced the transitions of life with grace? What if we stopped looking back, trying to return to a version of ourselves that no longer exists and instead looked ahead with compassion and curiosity, embracing who we are becoming?

Ageing is a real privilege. Not everyone gets to do it. The body may change, but we don't have to wither away. We have learned many tools through this book to stay flexible in mind, body and spirit, to keep learning, adapting to and loving life. The real question is not whether it's possible, but whether you are willing to believe it, and act accordingly. When you bring together the threads of wisdom, rhythm, nourishment and self-trust, something profound happens to your well-being.

In the quest to find ever-lasting youth through technological advances, we seem to have strayed away from the profound wisdom that once guided us. Our ancestors knew the value of nature's rhythm and that wisdom still lives through us, in our bones, in our blood, in our breath. *Rasāyana* opens the pathways back to that remembrance. We're guided to nourish and replenish instead of restricting and depleting, to align instead of hustle, to age with intention, not fear.

How we live shapes how we age. Our mindset, daily habits, emotions, purpose and diet are the building blocks of vitality. We should not view ageing as a condition to pathologise but rather a process we can *all* master.

You do not need to wait for the signs of decline to start making change. Wherever you are, you can start. *Now* is the only moment that is real and now is always the perfect time to invest in your future self. True well-being will not be found in a prescription but through pause. So, pause. Reflect. No matter your age, it's your birthright to reclaim your health with agency and out of deep love for life. In doing so, you honour yourself, those who came before you and those who will follow. This isn't the end, it's a sacred return.

पश्येम शरदः शतम् । जीवेम शरदः शतम् । बुध्येम शरदः शतम् ॥

paśyema śaradaḥ śatam |
jīvema śaradaḥ śatam |
budhyema śaradaḥ śatam ||

'May we see a hundred autumns; may we live for a hundred autumns; may we remain mentally awake.'
Atharva Veda, 19.67.1–3

Sanskrit glossary

Abhyanga	Warm oil body massage
Ācārya	A sage, teacher or master of Vedic traditions
***Ācārya* Caraka**	Ancient *Āyurvedic* physician and author of the *Caraka Saṃhitā*
***Ācārya* Suśruta**	Ancient *Āyurvedic* surgeon and author of the *Suśruta Saṃhitā*
Ādhyātmika	Relating to the inner self; spiritual or internal in nature
Advaita Vedānta	A non-dualistic school of Indian philosophy that teaches the unity of the self (*ātman*) with the ultimate reality (*brahman*)
Agni	The element of fire or digestive/metabolic fire in the body
Āhāra	Nourishment or food; one of the three pillars of health in *Āyurveda*
Āhāra rasa	The end product of digested food
Āma	Improperly digested metabolic residue from weak *agni*; it underlies many diseases and is commonly referred to as 'toxins'
Āma pācana	Digesting and clearing accumulated toxins from the body
Amla	Sour taste
Anitya	Impermanence/transience

Añjali	An *Āyurvedic* volumetric measure for food. One *añjali* equals the volume of palms cupped together
Anupāna	A substance that serves as a medium to carry herbs to the body tissues. For example, ghee, milk and water
Ārtava	Female reproductive tissue; associated with menstrual health
Ārtha	1. The object of the senses (sound, touch, form, taste, smell) 2. Material prosperity or wealth; one of the four *purushārthas* or aims of life
Āsana	Yoga posture or pose
Āśramas	The four stages of life: *brahmacharya* (student), *gṛhastha* (householder), *vānaprastha* (forest dweller) and *sannyāsa* (renunciate)
Ashtāṅga Hṛdaya	An authoritative and influential text of *Āyurveda* written by Sage Vāgbhaṭa
Asthi dhātu	Bone tissue
Āyurveda	The ancient system of healing and natural medicine known as the science of life
Bala	Physical and mental strength/vitality
Bhūtāgni	The digestive fire that transforms *āhāra rasa* into the five elements (*mahābhūtas* - space, air, fire, water and earth)
Brahma muhūrta	The auspicious early morning time (about 1.5 hours before sunrise), which is ideal for spiritual practices
Brahmacharya	Celibacy or correct use of sexual energy; also refers to the student stage of life and a life of discipline
Bṛṃhaṇa	A substance, process or treatment that tonifies, builds and nourishes the body; anabolic in nature
Caraka	A sage (*Ṛṣi & Ācārya*) of the *Āyurvedic* system of medicine and lifestyle. He is famous for writing the medical treatise called the *Caraka Saṃhitā*
Chakra	An Anglicised form of the Sanskrit word for 'wheel' or 'vortex'. There are seven primary energetic vortices (or nerve plexus centres) that form part of the energetic body found near the spinal cord, where a number of subtle energy channels known as *nādīs* intersect

Cyavanaprāśa	A classic *Āyurvedic* herbal jam made with *amalaki* and *rasāyana* herbs, traditionally used for rejuvenation (often styled as Chyawanprash)
Dharma	Righteous duty or one's true path; an essential aim of life
Dhātu kṣaya	Depletion of bodily tissues
Dhātu parināma	The sequential transformation process of tissues in *Āyurveda*; how one *dhātu* nourishes the next
Dhātus	The seven fundamental body constituents that build, nourish and sustain the living body – often translated as '*tissues*' though defined by function than anatomy
Dhātusāmya	Dynamic harmony of tissues and functions
Dhātvagni	The digestive fire located in the body tissue
Dhyāna	Act of meditation and contemplation
Dinacaryā	*Āyurvedic* daily health regimen
Dīpana	Natural substances that kindle the digestive fire and strengthen appetite
Doṣa	A natural energy force in the body, of which there are three: *vāta*, *pittā* and *kapha*. *Doṣas* are responsible for all functions in the body and each has distinct characteristics, making up your unique constitution
Ekādaśī	Eleventh day of the lunar cycle (both waxing and waning) – ideal day for fasting
Garśana	Dry body brushing
Ghee	Clarified butter
Gṛhastha	Householder stage of life
Guṇa	1. The quality or attribute of a food, spice or herb 2. Referring to the quality of the mind
Indriya	A faculty of perception (sense organ)
Jala	The element of water
Jarā	Ageing supported in *Āyurveda* through *rasāyana*
Jarāvasthā	The ageing stage of life and one's state – physical, emotional and spiritual
Jaṭharāgni	Fire responsible for digestion and absorption of food
Jyotiṣa	Vedic astrology
Kāla	Time/natural cycles
Kāma	Desire, pleasure and enjoyment; one of the four *purushārthas*

Kapālabhāti	Yogic breathing technique (Skull Shining Breath)
Kapha	*Kapha* is the *doṣa* that governs structure and cohesiveness. *Kapha* is predominated by the earth and water elements. It is heavy, slow, cool, oily, smooth, dense, soft, stable and cloudy
Karma	1. The action of a substance on the body 2. Daily choices and actions, both past and present
Kaṣāya	Astringent taste
Kaṭu	Pungent taste
Kavala	Ancient oral hygiene technique known as oil pulling (swishing of oil/liquid in the mouth).
Kāya-kalpa	Ancient *Āyurvedic* rejuvenation therapy for body transformation and longevity
Khichdi	A dish made of rice and mung dal
Kuti praveśikā	A type of intensive *Kāya Kalpa* therapy involving isolation for deep rejuvenation
Laṅghana	Reduction and lightening therapies usually referring to fasting and detoxification; catabolic in nature
Lavana	Salty taste
Likhita japa	A devotional practice of writing a mantra repeatedly as meditation
Līlā	Divine play/playfulness
Madhura	Sweet taste
Malas	The waste products that are excreted out of the body, primarily through urine, faeces and sweat
Māṃsa	Muscle tissue
Manas	The mind
Mandāgni	Slow or weakened state of the digestive fire. Can be considered hypometabolism
Mantra	Sacred words or phrases that are recited aloud or in silence. They hold a vibration in the body
Marma	Energy points on the surface of the body that correlate to subtle channels of the body. They relate to specific organs, channels and energies. Used in healing treatments
Mauna	Silence or conscious silence
Medhya rasāyana	*Rasāyana* herbs that enhance cognitive function and mental clarity
Mokṣa	Liberation or spiritual freedom; the ultimate aim of life

Mudrā	A hand sign or gesture commonly practised in yoga
Mūrchita taila	Cured sesame oil – a heat-processed oil in which impurities are removed, making it lighter, more stable and penetrative. Used for massage and oil pulling
Nādī	A tubular channel of the physical or subtle body; for example, a vein or artery
Nādī Śodhana	Yogic breathing technique (alternate nostril breath)
Nasya	The therapeutic administration of medicated oil in the nasal passages to clear imbalanced *doṣas* in the ear, nose and throat area. One of the five purification treatments
***Neti* pot**	A small watering can-style pot used for nasal cleansing
Nidrā	Sleep; one of the three pillars of health in *Āyurveda*
Ojas	The subtle energy of *kapha*. The end product when tissue formation is complete, and the foundation of our immune system
Pācana	A substance that neutralises toxins and *āma* in the body
Pañca kośas/ kośas	The five sheaths or layers of human existence
Pañca mahābhūtas	The five great elements of *ākāśa* (ether), *vayu* (air), *tejas* (fire), *jala* (water), *pṛthvī* (earth)
Pañcakarma	Five purification treatments that fall under *śodhana* therapies
Pittā	*Pittā* is the *doṣa* that governs all digestion and transformation in the body. Predominated by the fire and water elements, it is light, penetrating, hot, oily, liquid and spreading
Prakṛti	Your mind/body constitution derived from a unique composition of *vāta, pittā* and *kapha*
Prāṇa	The subtle energy of *vāta*. Considered the life-force energy associated with incoming energy from breath, and also water and food
Prajñāparādha	Acting against better judgment due to error of the intellect
Prāṇāyāma	A series of yogic breathing techniques
Pṛthvī	The element of earth
Purusha	The consciousness or the soul

Purushārthas	The four goals of human life: *dharma*, *ārtha*, *kāma* and *mokṣa*
Rajas	The quality of action, energy and stimulation that generates sensual reaction, pleasure and pain
Rakta	Blood tissue
Rasa	1. The taste of a food (sweet, sour, salty, bitter, pungent, astringent) 2. The name of the plasma tissue (***rasa dhātu***)
Rasāyana	Science of rejuvenation, or a substance that nourishes, heals and rejuvenates, acting as a tonic for the entire body (cells, tissues and organs)
Ṛṣi (Rishi)	An ancient seer or revealer of Vedic wisdom
Ṛtucaryā	Seasonal regimen according to the natural cycle of the seasons
Sadvṛtta	Ethical living and right conduct
Samāgni	Balanced and resilient state of digestion
Saṃsāra	The cycle of birth, death and rebirth; associated with worldly attachments
Saṃskāra	Mental impressions formed by past actions and experiences
Saṅkalpa	A heartfelt intention or vow used in healing and spiritual practices
Sannyāsa	A life phase of renunciation
Sanskrit	One of the oldest ancient languages, from which Hindi derives
Sapta dhātu	Seven sustaining body tissues – *See Dhātus*
Ṣaṭkarma	Six cleansing actions in Haṭha Yoga
Satsaṅga	In the company of truth (with community)
Sattva	The quality of purity that gives rise to lightness, luminosity and harmony in the mind and body; palliative therapies
Sattvavajaya	Mastery of the mind through psycho-spiritual therapy and mental discipline
Śīta	Cold quality
'So Hum'	A meditative mantra meaning 'I am That'; aligns self with universal consciousness
Soma	A divine elixir in Vedic tradition associated with rejuvenation and bliss
Srotas	The physical and subtle channels of the body
Śukra	Male reproductive tissue

Sūrya Namaskāra	Sun Salutation; a yoga sequence honouring the sun and energising the body
Suśruta	A sage (*Ṛṣi & Ācārya*) of the *Āyurvedic* system of medicine and surgery. He is known as the father of surgery, writing the medical treatise, the *Suśruta Samhita*
Svadharma	One's personal *dharma* or inner calling
Svādhyāya	Self-study or self-development
Svastha	A balanced state of health
Svāsthavṛtta	The theory and practice of preventative health using daily and seasonal regimens
Svasthya	Health; literally 'to be established in the self'
Svedana	*Āyurvedic* sweating therapy for detoxification and circulation
Tamas	The mental quality of dullness, darkness and inertia
Tat tvam asi	'Thou art That'; a teaching expressing oneness of individual and universal self
Tejas	The subtle form of *agni* or *pittā* in the body that governs intelligence, discernment and enthusiasm
Tikṣṇāgni	Acute, strong and intense state of digestive fire. Can be considered as hypermetabolism
Tikta	Bitter taste
Trāṭaka	Candle-gazing meditation practice
Tridoṣa	A combination of the three *doṣas*, *vāta*, *pittā* and *kapha*
Triphala	A traditional *Āyurvedic* compound of three fruits – *amalaki*, *haritaki* and *bibhitaki*. Its properties help to gently cleanse and detoxify the digestive tract, support regularity and nourish the tissues
Udvartana	An *Āyurvedic* massage with herbal powders for detox and fat metabolism
Upavāsa	Fasting or food abstinence used for cleansing and discipline
Uṣṇa	Hot, fiery or heating quality
Vānaprastha	The forest-dweller stage of life
Vāsanā	A karmic imprint or subconscious tendency influencing behaviour
Vastu	Vedic system of architecture based on sacred and spatial geometry

Vāta The *doṣa* primarily responsible for all movement and communication in the body. *Vāta* is predominated by the ether and air elements. It is light, cold, dry, rough, mobile, subtle and clear

Vayu The element of air

Veda(s) The earliest collection of ancient Indian scriptures. They consist of four bodies of wisdom including: *Ṛgveda*, *Sāmaveda*, *Yajurveda* and *Atharvaveda*

Vedic Belonging to the traditions of the Vedas

Vihāra Lifestyle activities

Vikṛti The imbalanced or current state of your health

Vipāka The post-digestive effect of a food substance experienced in the latter stages of digestion

Vīrya The heating or cooling potency of an ingredient in the process of digestion before *vipāka*

Viṣamāgni Irregular or unstable digestive fire

Vyādhi-kṣamatva Immunity/resistance to disease

Vyayāma Physical exercise that promotes strength, stability and flexibility

Yoga A collection of physical, mental and spiritual practices intended to transform and liberate the mind and body

References

Introduction

1 **the number of people aged 60 years and older:** World Health Organization (2020). United Nations Decade of Healthy Ageing: Plan of Action. Geneva: World Health Organization. Available at: https://cdn.who.int/media/docs/default-source/decade-of-healthy-ageing/decade-proposal-final-apr2020-en.pdf

Chapter 1

16 **wider research findings on ageing fears:** Pfizer Inc. (2014). *New Survey Reveals 87% of Americans have a Fear of Getting Old (FOGO).* [Press release] 15 July. Available at: https://www.pfizer.com/news/press-release/press-release-detail/fogo_new_survey_reveals_87_of_americans_have_a_fear_of_getting_old_fogo_results_show_top_fear_is_decline_in_physical_ability1 **and** AARP (2025). *How Views on Aging Look Across Generations*. [online] AARP Research. Available at: https://www.aarp.org/pri/topics/aging-experience/views-aging-across-generations/

16 **a US survey revealed that one in four adults:** Phelan, E.A., et al., 'Older adults' views of "successful aging"–how do they compare with researchers' definitions?' *Journal of the American Geriatrics Society*, 52(2), 2004, 211–216.

16 **raise real concerns about physical limitation:** Awang, H., et al., 'Understanding ageing: fear of chronic diseases later in life', *Journal of International Medical Research*, 46(1), January 2018, 175–184.

16 **Concerns about outliving savings:** Nelson, T.D., 'Ageism: Prejudice Against Our Feared Future Self', *Journal of Social Issues*, 61(2), 2005, 207–221.

16 Anxiety about death tends to peak: Ayalon, L., 'Perceived age discrimination: A precursor of depressive symptoms and functional decline', *Journals of Gerontology: Series B*, 75(3), 2020, 526–535.

17 our modern lifestyles are accelerating biological ageing and decline: Chaudhary, M.R., et al., 'Aging, oxidative stress and degenerative diseases: mechanisms, complications and emerging therapeutic strategies', *Biogerontology*, 24(5), October 2023, 609–662.

23 'All that we are is the result of what we have thought': Muller, M., *Buddhist Texts From Japan* (Kessinger Publishing, 2009 [1881])

23 One compelling example is the Counterclockwise study: Langer, E.J., *Counterclockwise: Mindful Health and the Power of Possibility* (Ballantine Books, 2009).

24 Dan Buettner's Blue Zones research: Buettner, Dan. *The Blue Zones: Lessons for Living Longer from the People Who've Lived the Longest.* Washington, D.C.: National Geographic, 2008.

Chapter 2

26 potential to live healthily beyond 100 years: Dong, X., Milholland, B. and Vijg, J., 'Evidence for a limit to human lifespan', *Nature*, 538(7624), 13 October 2016, 257–259.

27 once seen mostly in the elderly: Ghosh, S., et al., 'Sedentary lifestyle with increased risk of obesity in urban adult academic professionals: an epidemiological study in West Bengal, India', *Scientific Reports*, 13(1), 25 March 2023, 4895.

27 overuse of synthetic medicines: Schmauck-Medina, T., et al., 'New hallmarks of ageing: a 2022 Copenhagen ageing meeting summary', *Aging (Albany NY)*, 14(16), 29 August 2022, 6829–6839.

29 The World Health Organization defines healthy ageing: World Health Organization (2015). 'World Report on Ageing and Health'. Available at: https://www.who.int/publications/i/item/9789241565042

31 a booming industry projected to have reached $1.3 trillion by 2025: Global Wellness Institute (2022). 'Projected to Hit $817 Billion This Year, $1.3 Trillion in 2025: New Data on Wellness Tourism'. https://www.globalwellnessinstitute.org/

Chapter 4

59 living with a strong sense of purpose: Hill, P.L. and Turiano, N.A., 'Purpose in Life as a Predictor of Mortality Across Adulthood', *Psychological Science*, 25(7), 2014, 1482–1486. Available at: doi:10.1177/0956797614531799 **and** Cohen, R., et al., 'Purpose in Life and Proinflammatory Gene Expression in Older Adults', *Health Psychology*, 35(9), 2016, 125–131. Available at: doi:10.1037/hea0000316 **and** Alimujiang, A., et al., 'Association Between Life Purpose and Mortality Among US Adults Older Than 50 Years', *JAMA Network Open*, 2(5), 2019, e194270. Available at: doi:10.1001/jamanetworkopen.2019.4270 **and** Yu, L., et al., 'Purpose in Life and Sleep: A Study of Older Adults', *Sleep Health*, 8(4), 2022, 343–349. Available at: doi:10.1016/j.sleh.2022.03.005

61 As Maslow highlights in his Hierachy of Needs: McLeod, S., 'Maslow's Hierarchy Of Needs', *Simple Psychology*, October 2025. Available at: www.simplypsychology.org/maslow.html

62 people those who experience love, intimacy and belonging: Holt-Lunstad, J., Robles, T.F. and Sbarra, D.A., 'Advancing social connection as a public health priority in the United States', *American Psychologist*, 78(4), 2023, 575–589.

65 The Revd. Dr Michael Beckwith's four stages of consciousness: Beckwith, M.B., 2012. *Life Visioning: A Transformative Process for Activating Your Unique Gifts and Highest Potential.* St Martin's Publishing Group, Boulder, CO.

71 'The mystery of life is not a problem to be solved': van der Leeuw, J.J. (1928). *The Conquest of Illusion*. New York: A.A. Knopf.

71 The trouble is, you think you have time.': Kornfield, J. (1994). *Buddha's Little Instruction Book*. San Francisco: Bantam Books.

Chapter 5

82 improve insulin sensitivity, reduce inflammation and lower the risk of chronic diseases: Xiaoyu, W., Yuxin, X. and Li, L., 'The effects of different intermittent fasting regimens in people with type 2 diabetes: a network meta-analysis', *Frontiers in Nutrition*, 11, 25 January 2024, article 1325894. Available at: www.frontiersin.org/journals/nutrition/articles/10.3389/fnut.2024.1325894/full **and** Aamir, A.B., et al., 'Effects of intermittent fasting and caloric restriction on inflammatory biomarkers in individuals with obesity/overweight: A systematic review and meta-analysis of randomized controlled trials', *Obesity Reviews*, 26(1), January 2025, e13838.

82 unlock remarkable vitality and longevity across the Blue Zone communities: Buettner, D., 'Lessons From the Blue Zones: There is No Silver Bullet (or Magic Pill) for a Long, Healthy Life', *American Journal of Lifestyle Medicine*, 1 May 2025, 15598276251334310.

83 reduce insulin resistance and, over time, could lower type 2 diabetes risk: Rovira-Llopis, S. et al., 'Circadian alignment of food intake and glycaemic control by time-restricted eating: A systematic review and meta-analysis', *Reviews in Endocrine and Metabolic Disorders*, 25(2), April 2024, 325–337.

85 Emerging research in humans suggests that intermittent fasting: Bensalem, J., Teong, J., Schlaich, M.P., Ahern, A.L. and Markovic, T.P., 2025. Intermittent time-restricted eating may increase autophagic flux in humans: an exploratory analysis. *Journal of Physiology*, 603(10), 3019–3032.

Pillar 1

100 it can mute our mental clarity, drain energy and affect mood: Phillips-Beyer, A. et al., 'Meaningful Within-Patient Change on the Insomnia Daytime Symptoms and Impacts Questionnaire (IDSIQ): Analysis of Phase III Clinical Trial Data of Daridorexant', *Pharmaceutical Medicine*, 37(4), July 2023, 291–303. **and** Palagini, L. et al. 'Insomnia, poor sleep quality and perinatal suicidal risk:

A systematic review and meta-analysis', *Journal of Sleep Research*, 33(2), April 2024, e14000.

100 **echoed in neuroscience as the *glymphatic system*:** Dengler, V., Westphalen, K. and Koeppen, M., 'Disruption of Circadian Rhythms and Sleep in Critical Illness and its Impact on Innate Immunity', *Current Pharmaceutical Design*, 21(24), 2015, 3469–3476. **and** Fagiani, F. et al., 'Misalignment in circadian-regulated glymphatic clearance as a driver of neurodegeneration', *Alzheimer's & Dementia*, 19, 2023.

100 **Sleep timing strongly affects our metabolic health:** Chaput, J.P. et al., 'Sleep timing, sleep consistency, and health in adults: a systematic review', *Applied Physiology, Nutrition, and Metabolism*, 45(10 (Suppl. 2)), 2020, S232–S247.

101 **boosting serotonin by day and melatonin by night:** Ohashi, M. et al., 'Relationship between Circadian Phase Delay without Morning Light and Phase Advance by Bright Light Exposure the Following Morning', *Clocks Sleep*, 5(4), 23 October 2023, 615–626.

101 **is the least disruptive on melatonin production:** Ho Mien, I. et al., 'Effects of exposure to intermittent versus continuous red light on human circadian rhythms, melatonin suppression, and pupillary constriction', *PLoS One*, 9(5), 5 May 2014, e96532.

102 **cellular detox and the glymphatic system are most active:** Lee, S. et al., 'Contrast-enhanced MRI T1 Mapping for Quantitative Evaluation of Putative Dynamic Glymphatic Activity in the Human Brain in Sleep-Wake States', *Radiology*, 300(3), September 2021, 661–668.

102 **mimic the effects of chronic illnesses:** Buxton, O.M. et al., 'Sleep Restriction For One Week Reduces Insulin Sensitivity In Healthy Men Running title: Insufficient sleep and insulin sensitivity', *Diabetes*, 59(9), 2010, 2126–2133. **and** Pejovic, S. et al., 'Effects of recovery sleep after one work week of mild sleep restriction on interleukin-6 and cortisol secretion and daytime sleepiness and performance', *American Journal of Physiology – Endocrinology and Metabolism*, 305(7), 1 October 2013, E890-E896.

104 **choose dim, candle or red lighting:** Han, X., Zhou, E. and Liu, D., 'Electronic Media Use and Sleep Quality: Updated Systematic Review and Meta-Analysis', *Journal of Medical Internet Research*, 26, 23 April 2024, e48356.

Pillar 2

109 **up from an estimated less than 5 per cent two centuries ago:** Lee, J.H., Duster, M., Roberts, T. and Devinsky, O., 'United States Dietary Trends Since 1800: Lack of Association Between Saturated Fatty Acid Consumption and Non-communicable Diseases', *Frontiers in Nutrition*, 8,13 January 2022, 748847. **and** Baraldi, L.G., Martinez Steele, E., Canella, D.S. and Monteiro, C.A., 'Consumption of ultra-processed foods and associated sociodemographic factors in the USA between 2007 and 2012: evidence from a nationally representative cross-sectional study', *BMJ Open*, 8(3): 9 March 2018, e020574.

109 two-thirds of what children and teens consume: Archer, E., Hand, G.A. and Blair, S.N., 'Validity of U.S. nutritional surveillance: National Health and Nutrition Examination Survey caloric energy intake data, 1971-2010', *PLoS One*, 8(10), 9 October 2013, e76632. **and** National Institutes of Health, 'Highly processed foods form bulk of U.S. youths' diets', *NIH Research Matters*, 24 August 2021.

109 compared to those who eat the least: Taylor, V., 'Ultra-processed foods: how bad are they for your health?', British Heart Foundation, 24 March 2025. Available at: www.bhf.org.uk/informationsupport/heart-matters-magazine/news/behind-the-headlines/ultra-processed-foods

117 the most celebrated *rasāyana* fat with its sweet, unctuous, cooling and regenerative qualities: (*Caraka Saṃhitā*, Sūtrasthāna. 27.323)

118 Traditional ghee is said to support vision: (*Aṣṭāṅga Hṛdaya*, Sūtrasthāna 5.35).

119 studies show how omega-3 fatty acids: Ibrahim Mohialdeen Gubari, M., 'Effect of omega-3 fatty acid supplementation on markers of inflammation and endothelial function in patients with chronic heart disease: A systematic review and meta-analysis', *Cellular and Molecular Biology (Noisy-le-Grand)*, 70(6), 5 June 2024, 171–177. **and** Kim, J.Y., Kong, S.Y.J., Jung, E. and Cho, Y.S., 'Omega-3 Fatty Acids as Potential Predictors of Sudden Cardiac Death and Cardiovascular Mortality: A Systematic Review and Meta-Analysis', *Journal of Clinical Medicine*, 14(1), 25 December 2024, 26. **and** Kusy, B., Parzecka, K., Kucharczyk, P. and Szczepanik, K., 'Long-chain polyunsaturated fatty acids and brain functions – literature review', *Wiadomości Lekarskie*, 77(6), 2024, 1277–1283.

119 heals the blood-brain barrier and provides neuroprotection: Gorzynik-Debicka, M. et al., 'Neuroprotective Effects of Olive Oil: A Comprehensive Review of Antioxidant Properties', *Antioxidants*, 13(7), 2024, 795.

119 studies showing 28 per cent lower dementia mortality: Tessier, A.J. et al., 'Consumption of Olive Oil and Diet Quality and Risk of Dementia-Related Mortality', *JAMA Network Open*, 7(5), 2024.

123 many elders take honey daily: Monroe, L., 'Honey–A Sweet Secret to Longevity', *Blue Zones*, 22 September 2021. Available at: www.bluezones.com/2021/09/honey-a-sweet-secret-to-longevity/

124 Studies show that whole, unprocessed wheat: Roager, H.M et al., 'Whole grain-rich diet reduces body weight and systemic low-grade inflammation without inducing major changes to the gut microbiome: a randomised cross-over trial', *Gut*, 68(1), 83-93. 2019. https://doi.org/10.1136/gutjnl-2017-314786

129 Their polyphenols and essential oils neutralise free radicals: Opara, E.I. and Chohan, M. (2014), 'Culinary Herbs and Spices: Their Bioactive Properties, the Contribution of Polyphenols and the Challenges in Deducing Their True Health Benefits'. *International Journal of Molecular Sciences*, 15(10), 19183–19202. https://doi.org/10.3390/ijms151019183 **and** Rudrapal, M. et al. (2022). 'Dietary Polyphenols and Their Role in Oxidative Stress-Induced Human Diseases: Insights Into Protective Effects, Antioxidant Potentials and Mechanism(s) of Action', *Frontiers in Pharmacology*, 13, 806470. https://doi.org/10.3389/fphar.2022.806470

144 a telomerase-modulating agent: Sharma, R. and Martins, N., 'Telomeres, DNA Damage and Ageing: Potential Leads from Ayurvedic Rasāyana (Anti-Ageing) Drugs', *Journal of Clinical Medicine*, 9(8), 6 August 2020, 2544.

144 preserve cellular integrity and reduce oxidative stress: Gul, M. et al., 'Functional and Nutraceutical Significance of Amla (*Phyllanthus emblica L.*): A Review', *Antioxidants*, 11(5), 22 April 2022, 816.

144 *amalaki*... showing potential as a stem cell and telomerase activator: Guruprasad, K.P., Dash, S., Shivakumar, M.B. et al., 'Influence of *Amalaki Rasayana* on telomerase activity and telomere length in human blood mononuclear cells', *Journal of Ayurveda and Integrative Medicine*, 2017, 8(2). Available at: https://www.ncbi.nlm.nih.gov/pmc/articles/PMC5497001/

145 slows greying, restores glow: Chanvorachote, P. et al., 'Type I pro-collagen promoting and anti-collagenase activities of Phyllanthus emblica extract in mouse fibroblasts', *Journal of Cosmetic Science*, 60(4), pp. 395–403. 2009. Available at: https://pubmed.ncbi.nlm.nih.gov/19691935/ **and** Sangeetha, N. et al. 'Phyllanthus emblica: a comprehensive review of its phytochemical and therapeutic profile', *Frontiers in Pharmacology*, 14: 128861. 2023. doi: 10.3389/fphar.2023.128861. Available at: https://www.frontiersin.org/articles/10.3389/fphar.2023.128861/full

145 Strengthens *agni*, cools acidity, improves absorption: Kapoor, M.P., Suzuki, K., Timm, D., Ozeki, M. and Okubo, T. 'Clinical evaluation of *Emblica officinalis* Gaertn (Amla) in healthy human subjects: Health benefits and safety results from a randomized, double-blind, crossover placebo-controlled study', *Contemporary Clinical Trials Communications*, 17, p. 100499. 2019. doi: 10.1016/j.conctc.2019.100499.

145 Sharpens memory, may reduce LDL cholesterol and trigycerides supporting vascular circulation: Brown, P. D. S. and Ketter, N. 'Clinical effects of Emblica officinalis fruit consumption on cardiovascular disease risk factors: a systematic review and meta-analysis', *BMC Complementary Medicine and Therapies*, 23: 266. 2023. Available at: https://www.ncbi.nlm.nih.gov/pmc/articles/PMC10251691/

146 preclinical evidence suggesting it may influence stem-cell-related pathways and telomerase activity: Raguraman, V. and Subramaniam, J.R. (2016) 'Withania somnifera root extract enhances telomerase activity in the human HeLa cell line', Advances in Bioscience and Biotechnology, 7(4), pp. 199–204. doi:10.4236/abb.2016.74018 **and** Tripathi, A.K., Sardar, A., Rai, N., Rai, D., Girme, A., Sinha, S., Chutani, K., Hingorani, L., Mishra, P.R. and Trivedi, R. (2024) 'Withaferin A ameliorated the bone marrow fat content in obese male mice by favoring osteogenesis in bone marrow mesenchymal stem cells and preserving the bone mineral density', ACS Pharmacology & Translational Science, 7(9), pp. 2621–2636. doi:10.1021/acsptsci.3c00356

146 *Aśvagandhā* helps regulate cortisol and other stress hormones: Della Porta, M., Maier, J.A. and Cazzola, R. 'Effects of Withania somnifera on cortisol levels in stressed human subjects: A systematic review', *Nutrients*, 15(24), 5015. 2023. doi: 10.3390/nu15245015. Available at: https://doi.org/10.3390/nu15245015

146 *aśvagandhā* restores stamina and energy: Lee, D.H. et al., 'Withania somnifera Extract Enhances Energy Expenditure via Improving Mitochondrial Function in Adipose Tissue and Skeletal Muscle', *Nutrients*, 12(2), 7 February 2020, 431. **and** Wankhede, S. et al., 'Examining the Effect of *Withania somnifera* Supplementation on Muscle Strength and Recovery: A Randomized Controlled Trial', *Journal of the International Society of Sports Nutrition*, 12, 25 November 2015, 43.

146 *Aśvagandhā* enhances memory, focus and neuroplasticity: Konar, A. and Thakur, M.K., 'Cellular and Molecular Targets Underpinning Memory Enhancement by Ashwagandha', in *Neuroprotective Natural Products: Clinical Aspects and Mode of Action* (Springer, 2017).

146 especially soothing for insomnia, stress-induced fatigue and tension: Langade, D., Kanchi, S., Salve, J., Debnath, K. and Ambegaokar, D. 'Efficacy and Safety of Ashwagandha (*Withania somnifera* [L.] Dunal) Root Extract in Insomnia and Anxiety: A Double-Blind, Randomized, Placebo-Controlled Study', *Cureus*, 11(9): e5797. 2019. doi: 10.7759/cureus.5797.

146 *Aśvagandhā* helps reduce inflammation and oxidative stress: KrishnaRaju, A.V., Shukla, A. Chandra, A. et al. (2023), 'Efficacy and anti-inflammatory activity of Ashwagandha (Withania somnifera [L.] Dunal) root extract: mechanistic insights and therapeutic potential', *Journal of Inflammation Research*, 16, pp. 3795–3810. doi: 10.2147/JIR.S853643. Available at: https://www.dovepress.com/article_download/85398

147 Studies on *bibhitaki* point to its anti-inflammatory, antiviral and antimicrobial properties: Jayesh, K. et al., '*Terminalia bellirica* (Gaertn.) Roxb Fruit Exerts Anti-Inflammatory Effect via Regulating Arachidonic Acid Pathway and Pro-Inflammatory Cytokines in Lipopolysaccharide-Induced RAW 264.7 Macrophages', *Inflammopharmacology*, 12 July 2018. **and** Das, G. et al., 'Plants of the Genus *Terminalia*: An Insight on Its Biological Potentials, Pre-Clinical and Clinical Studies', *Frontiers in Pharmacology*, 11, 8 October 2020, 561248. **and** Tiwana, G. et al., 'Phytochemical Analysis and Antimicrobial Activity of *Terminalia bellirica* (Gaertn.) Roxb. and *Terminalia chebula* Retz. Fruit Extracts Against Gastrointestinal Pathogens: Enhancing Antibiotic Efficacy', *Microorganisms*, 12(12), 22 December 2024, 2664.

147 modern studies show it protects the intestinal lining and promotes regular bowel function: Li, Y.-Y. et al., '*Terminalia bellirica* fruit extract alleviates DSS-induced ulcerative colitis by regulating gut microbiota, inflammatory mediators, and cytokines', *Frontiers in Cellular and Infection Microbiology*, 12, 1054205. 2023. doi: 10.3389/fcimb.2022.1054205.

148 research pointing to its neuroprotective effects: Rajaduraivelpandian, P.B. et al., 'The Cognitive-Enhancing Properties of the Aqueous Extract from the fruit of *Terminalia bellirica* (Gaertn.) Roxb.', *Biomedical and Pharmacology Journal*, 2024.

148 clinically proven useful for mental illness (*unmadahara*): Calabrese, C. et al., 'Effects of a Standardized *Bacopa monnieri* Extract on Cognitive Performance, Anxiety, and Depression in the Elderly: A Randomized, Double-Blind, Placebo-Controlled Trial', *Journal of Alternative and Complementary Medicine*, 14(6), 2008, 707–713.

149 protects against age-related cognitive decline and neuroinflammation: McPhee, G.M. et al., 'The Neurocognitive Effects of *Bacopa monnieri* and Cognitive Training on Markers of Brain Microstructure in Healthy Older Adults', *Frontiers in Aging Neuroscience*, 13, 22 February 2021, 638109.

149 helping to reduce anxiety and elevate mood: Benson, S. et al., 'An Acute, Double-Blind, Placebo-Controlled Cross-Over Study of 320 mg and 640 mg Doses of *Bacopa monnieri* (CDRI 08) on Multitasking Stress Reactivity and Mood', *Phytotherapy Research*, 28(4), April 2014, 551–559. **and** Mathur, D. et al., 'The Molecular Links of Re-Emerging Therapy: A Review of Evidence of Brahmi (*Bacopa monniera*)', *Frontiers in Pharmacology*, 7, 4 March 2016, 44.

149 *brahmi* protects DNA from oxidative stress-induced damage: Nopparat, J. et al., 'Exploring the Excellence of Commercial Brahmi Products from Thai Online Markets: Unraveling Phytochemical Contents, Antioxidant Properties and DNA Damage Protection', *Heliyon*, 10(2), 17 January 2024, e24509.

149 *Brahmi* also reduces systemic inflammation: Nemetchek, M.D. et al., 'The Ayurvedic Plant *Bacopa monnieri* Inhibits Inflammatory Pathways in the Brain', *Journal of Ethnopharmacology*, 197, 2 February 2017, 92–100.

149 helping to minimise fine lines and promote a healthy complexion: Hwang, E., Lee, S., Kim, Y., Park, S. and Boo, Y. (2023), '*Bacopa monnieri* extract improves skin fibroblast activity and collagen production through antioxidant mechanisms', *Nutrients*, 17(11), 1939. https://doi.org/10.3390/nu17111939

149 Modern research shows that *Brahmi* modulates cytokines and immune pathways: Roy, S., Shanmugam, G., Rakshit, S., Pradeep, R., George, M. and Sarkar, K. (2024), 'Exploring the immunomodulatory potential of Brahmi (Bacopa monnieri) in the treatment of invasive ductal carcinoma', *Medical Oncology*, 41(5): 115. doi:10.1007/s12032-024-02365-x **and** Bhawane, B.S. et al., 'Brahmi Face Mist for Skin Rejuvenation and Protection', *International Journal for Multidisciplinary Research (IJFMR)*, 7(2), 2025, Article IJFMR250241691.

150 *Guḍūcī* … reducing chronic inflammation while increasing resistance to viral infections: Yates, C.R., Bruno, E.J. and Yates, M.E.D., '*Tinospora cordifolia*: A Review of Its Immunomodulatory Properties', *Journal of Dietary Supplements*, 19(2), 2022, 271–285. **and** Sharma, U. et al., 'Immunomodulatory Active Compounds from *Tinospora cordifolia*', *Journal of Ethnopharmacology*, 141(3), 14 June 2012, 918–926.

151 while shielding the brain from oxidative stress and cognitive decline: Jamadagni, S.B. et al., 'Amelioration of AlC3l$_3$-Induced Memory Loss in Rats by an Aqueous Extract of Guduchi, a *Medhya Rasāyana*', *Pharmacognosy Magazine*, 19, 2023, 231–243. **and** Mittal,

S., Mishra, S. and Malviya, K., 'A Comprehensive Review on the Study of *Medhya Rasāyana* in Mental Disorders', *International Ayurvedic Medical Journal*, 2025.

152 *Haritaki* gently regulates elimination: Singh, R.P., Sharma, A., Gupta, V. and Nag, T. (2013), 'A comparative evaluation of intestinal transit time of two dosage forms of *Terminalia chebula* Retz. (Churna & Vati) in mice', *Journal of Ayurveda & Integrative Medicine*, 4(2), pp. 82–88. doi:10.1016/j.jaim.2013.04.001

152 Research shows it supports gut motility and helps protect the intestinal mucosa: Dong, W.-R., Zhang, T., Zhao, Y.-Z., Li, Z., Zhang, Z., Yu, B. and et al. (2023), 'Ethyl acetate extract of *Terminalia chebula* alleviates DSS-induced ulcerative colitis in C57BL/6 mice via antioxidant and anti-inflammatory mechanisms', *Frontiers in Pharmacology*, 14, 1229772. doi:10.3389/fphar.2023.122977

152 *haritaki* protects cells from oxidative stress and inflammation: Khazani, H. et al., '*Terminalia chebula* Attenuates Restraint Stress-Induced Memory Impairment and Synaptic Loss in the Dentate Gyrus of the Hippocampus and the Basolateral and Central Nuclei of the Amygdala by Inhibiting Oxidative Damage', *Brain Research Bulletin*, 213, July 2024, 110975. **and** Ekambaram, S.P. et al., 'Modulation of NF-κB and MAPK Signalling Pathways by Hydrolysable Tannin Fraction from *Terminalia chebula* Fruits Contributes to Its Anti-Inflammatory Action in RAW 264.7 Cells', *Journal of Pharmacy and Pharmacology*, 74(5), 20 May 2022, 718–729.

152 protects brain tissue from oxidative damage: Gao, H. et al., 'The Potential of *Terminalia chebula* in Alleviating Mild Cognitive Impairment: A Review', *Frontiers in Pharmacology*, 15, 18 October 2024, 1484040.

153 hot flushes, dryness and mood fluctuations: Gudise, V.S., Dasari, M.P. and Kuricheti, S.S.K., 'Efficacy and Safety of Shatavari Root Extract for the Management of Menopausal Symptoms: A Double-Blind, Multicenter, Randomized Controlled Trial', *Cureus*, 16(4), 8 April 2024, e57879.

153 *Śatāvarī* helps the body adapt to stress, eases fatigue and supports immune balance: Gautam, M., Diwanay, et al. (2009), 'Immunomodulatory activity of Asparagus racemosus on systemic Th1/Th2 immunity in SRBC sensitized animals', *Journal of Ethnopharmacology*, 121(3), 541–547. https://doi.org/10.1016/j.jep.2008.11.023

153 regulates healthy digestion: Bhatnagar, M., Sisodia, S.S. and Bhatnagar, R. (2005), 'Antiulcer and antioxidant activity of *Asparagus racemosus* Willd. root extract in rats', *Journal of Herbal Pharmacotherapy*, 5(3), pp. 19–33. doi:10.1300/J157v05n03_03

153 help regulate blood sugar: Sharma, R., Amin, H., Galib, and Prajapati, P.K. (2014), 'Therapeutic potential of *Asparagus racemosus* in diabetes mellitus: An experimental study', *Ancient Science of Life*, 33(4), pp. 183–188. doi:10.4103/0257-7941.146612.

153 and cholesterol levels: Visavadiya, N.P. and Narasimhacharya, A.V.R.L. (2009), 'Hypocholesterolemic and antioxidant effects of *Asparagus racemosus* (Shatavari) root powder in hypercholesteremic rats', *Indian*

Journal of Pharmacology, 41(6), pp. 294–298. doi:10.4103/0253-7613.59932.

153 especially during hormonal transitions: Singh, N. et al., 'Adaptogenic Property of *Asparagus racemosus*: Future Trends and Prospects', *Heliyon*, 9(4), 1 April 2023, e14932.

156 *triphala* ... protects against oxidative stress and enhances *ojas* and immune resilience: Varma, S.R. et al., 2016, 'Protective Effects of Triphala on Dermal Fibroblasts and Human Keratinocytes', *PLOS ONE*, 11(1), e0145921. doi:10.1371/journal.pone.0145921. **and** Srikumar, R., Parthasarathy, N.J., Manikandan, S., Narayanan, G.S. and Sheeladevi, R., 2006, 'Effect of Triphala on oxidative stress and on cell-mediated immune response against noise stress in rats', *Molecular & Cellular Biochemistry*, 283(1–2), pp. 67–74. doi:10.1007/s11010-006-2271-0.

156 rich in antioxidants and has anti-inflammatory, antibacterial and antiviral properties: Bairwa, V.K., Kashyap, A. K., Meena, P. and Jain, B.P. (2025), 'Triphala's characteristics and potential therapeutic uses in modern health', *International Journal of Physiology, Pathophysiology and Pharmacology*, 17(2), 19-36. https://doi.org/10.62347/OBSS5026

157 *Cyavanaprāśa* ... enhances digestion, assimilation and metabolism while building strength, stamina and muscle tone: Sharma, R., Martins, N., Kuca, K., Chaudhary, A., Kabra, A., Rao, M.M. and Prajapati, P.K. (2019), 'Chyawanprash: A Traditional Indian Bioactive Health Supplement', *Biomolecules*, 9(5), 161. https://doi.org/10.3390/biom9050161

Pillar 4

161 even after accounting for physical activity levels: Biswas, A. et al., 'Sedentary Time and Cardiovascular Risk in Adults: A Systematic Review and Meta-Analysis', *Annals of Internal Medicine*, 162(2), 2015, 123–132. **and** Wu, J., Zhang, H., Yang, L. et al. (2022), 'Sedentary time and the risk of metabolic syndrome: A systematic review and dose-response meta-analysis', Obesity, 30(10), pp. 1900–1915. doi: 10.1002/oby.23526 **and** Bell, J.A., Hamer, M., Sabia, S., et al. (2014), 'Combined effect of physical activity and leisure time sitting on the long-term risk of obesity and metabolic risk factor clustering', *Diabetologia*, 57(8), pp. 1570–1581. doi: 10.1007/s00125-014-3279-8 **and** Alzahrani, H., Alshehri, A.A., et al. (2022), 'The association between sedentary behavior and low back pain in adults: a systematic review and meta-analysis of longitudinal studies', PeerJ, 10, p. e13127. doi: 10.7717/peerj.13127

161 supports holistic health by improving mood: Weinstein, A.A. et al., 'Affective Responses to Acute Exercise: A Meta-Analysis of the Potential Beneficial Effects of a Single Bout of Exercise on General Mood, Anxiety, and Depressive Symptoms', *Psychosomatic Medicine*, 86(6), July–August 2024, 486–497.

161 lowering cortisol levels: Zhao, L. and Mohammad, M., 'Testosterone and Cortisol Responses to ß-Hydroxy ß-Methylbutyrate Consumption and Exercise: A Meta-Analysis', *Food Science & Nutrition*, 10(9), 15 April 2022, 2815–2824.

161 and enhancing neuroplasticity: Kaagman, D.G.M. et al., 'Effects and Mechanisms of Exercise on Brain-Derived Neurotrophic Factor (BDNF) Levels and Clinical Outcomes in People with Parkinson's Disease: A Systematic Review and Meta-Analysis', *Brain Sciences*, 14(3), 21 February 2024, 194.

161 contributes to mental health and longevity: Duncan, M.J. et al., 'The Associations Between Physical Activity, Sedentary Behaviour, and Sleep with Mortality and Incident Cardiovascular Disease, Cancer, Diabetes and Mental Health in Adults: A Systematic Review and Meta-Analysis of Prospective Cohort Studies', *Journal of Active Sedentary and Sleep Behaviour*, 2(1), 4 September 2023, 19.

163 Studies on NEAT (Non-Exercise Activity Thermogenesis) highlight that incidental movement throughout the day: Levine, J.A. (2002), 'Non-exercise activity thermogenesis (NEAT)', *Best Practice & Research Clinical Endocrinology & Metabolism*, 16(4), 679–702. https://doi.org/10.1053/beem.2002.0227

164 especially for less active individuals: Del Pozo Cruz, B. et al., 'Light-Intensity Physical Activity and Life Expectancy: National Health and Nutrition Survey', *American Journal of Preventive Medicine*, 61(3), September 2021, 428–433.

164 just 10 to 15 minutes: Wen, C.P., Wai, J.P.M., Tsai, M.K., Yang, Y.C., Cheng, T.Y.D., Lee, M.C., Chan, H.T., Tsao, C.K., Tsai, S.P. and Wu, X. (2011), 'Minimum amount of physical activity for reduced mortality and extended life expectancy: a prospective cohort study', *The Lancet*, 378(9798), 1244–1253. https://doi.org/10.1016/S0140-6736(11)60749-6

166 Yoga has been proven to reduce markers of inflammation: Mishra, B. et al., 'Effectiveness of Yoga in Modulating Markers of Immunity and Inflammation: A Systematic Review and Meta-Analysis', *Cureus*, 16(4), 3 April 2024, e57541.

166 improve flexibility and support mental well-being: Ko, K.Y., Kwok, Z.C.M. and Chan, H.Y., 'Effects of Yoga on Physical and Psychological Health Among Community-Dwelling Older Adults: A Systematic Review and Meta-Analysis', *International Journal of Older People Nursing*, 18(5), September 2023, e12562.

166 top 10 yoga postures for pro-ageing: Postures selected from *Hatha Yoga Pradipika, Shiva Saṃhitā* and *Gheranda Saṃhitā.*

171 Getting up and down from the floor regularly has even been linked to greater mobility and longevity: de Brito, L.B.B., Ricardo, D.R., de Araújo, D.S.M.S., Ramos, P.S., Myers, J. and de Araújo, C.G.S. (2014), 'Ability to sit and rise from the floor as a predictor of all-cause mortality', *European Journal of Preventive Cardiology*, 21(7), 892–898. https://doi.org/10.1177/2047487312471759

173 the first five years after menopause: Thornton, M.J., 'Estrogens and Aging Skin', *Dermatoendocrinology*, 5(2), 2013, 264–270.

173 more sensitive and slower to heal: Horng, H.C., Chang, W.H., Yeh, C.C. et al., 'Estrogen Effects on Wound Healing', *International Journal of Molecular Sciences*, 18(11), 3 November 2017, 2325.

173 also impacts muscle and bone density: Hou, C.H., Hsieh, T.J. and Chou, M.C., 'Association Between Lumbar Muscle Size and Bone Mineral Density in Nonfractured Postmenopausal Women With and Without Osteoporosis', *Menopause*, 31(4), 2024, 282–287.

173 free radical damage and break down collagen: Hegde, A.N., Duke, L.M., Timm, L.E. and Nobles, H., 'The Proteasome and Ageing', *Subcellular Biochemistry*, 102, 2023, 99–112.

173 makes them more prone to damage: Danby, F.W., 'Nutrition and Aging Skin: Sugar and Glycation', *Clinics in Dermatology*, 28(4), July–August 2010, 409–411.

180 show oestrogen-like activity: National Cancer Institute, 'Antiperspirants and Breast Cancer Risk – Fact Sheet', *U.S. Department of Health and Human Services, National Institutes of Health*, 18 August 2022.

180 the damaging effects of air pollution: van der Wall, E.E., 'Air Pollution: 6.6 Million Premature Deaths in 2050!', *Netherlands Heart Journal*, 23(12), December 2015, 557–558.

186 concerns for both human health and marine ecosystems: Nguyen, T.H. and Vu, H.N., 'The Banned Sunscreen Ingredients and Their Impact on Human Health and the Environment', *Cureus*, 12(2), 2020, e7011. **and** Downs, C.A. et al., 'Toxicopathological Effects of the Sunscreen UV Filter, Oxybenzone (Benzophenone-3), on Coral Planulae and Cultured Primary Cells and Its Environmental Contamination in Hawaii and the U.S. Virgin Islands', *Archives of Environmental Contamination and Toxicology*, 70(2), February 2016, 265–288. 30/31.

187 Modern research continues to explore these botanicals: Moy, R.L. and Levenson, C. (2017), 'Sandalwood Album Oil as a Botanical Therapeutic in Dermatology', *The Journal of Clinical and Aesthetic Dermatology*, 10(10), pp. 34–39. Available at: https://www.ncbi.nlm.nih.gov/pmc/articles/PMC5749697/ **and** Hoffmann, J., Gendrisch, F., Schempp, C.M. and Wölfle, U. (2020), 'New Herbal Biomedicines for the Topical Treatment of Dermatological Disorders', *Biomolecules*, 10(2), p. 264. doi:10.3390/biom10020264.

Pillar 5

192 The *Hatha Yoga Pradipika* teaches that slow breathing increases vitality: Coats, A.J. Adamopoulos, S., Radaelli, A., McCance, A., Meyer, T.E. Bernardi, L., and Giannuzzi, P. (2002), 'Slow breathing increases arterial baroreflex sensitivity in patients with chronic heart failure', *Circulation*, 105(2), 143–145. DOI: https://doi.org/10.1161/hc0202.103311

193 softening extreme moods: Shah, M.R. and Kothari, P.H., 'Effects of Nadi-Shodhana Pranayama on Depression, Anxiety, Stress and Peak Expiratory Flow Rate in Post-CABG Patients: Experimental Study', *International Journal of Health Sciences Research*, 9(10), 2019, 40–45. **and** Ghiya, S. (2017), 'Alternate nostril breathing: A systematic review of clinical trials', *International Journal of Research in Ayurveda and Pharmacy*, 8(Suppl 3), pp. 1–9. doi:10.7897/2277-4343.083201

196 even how well our cells regenerate: Dasanayaka, N.N., Sirisena, N.D. and Samaranayake, N., 'Associations of Meditation with Telomere Dynamics: A Case-Control Study in Healthy Adults', *Frontiers in Psychology*, 14, 2023, 1222863. **and** Linz, R., Singer, T. and Engert, V., 'Interactions of Momentary Thought Content and Subjective Stress Predict Cortisol Fluctuations in a Daily Life Experience Sampling Study', *Scientific Reports*, 8, 2018, 15462.

196 fuelling inflammation, disrupting cortisol rhythms and depleting our emotional reserves: Nealis, L.J. et al. (2020), 'Self-critical perfectionism, depressive symptoms, and HPA-axis dysregulation: testing emotional and physiological stress reactivity', *Journal of Psychopathology and Behavioral Assessment*, 42, pp. 509–523. doi: 10.1007/s10862-020-09793-9 **and** Szabo, Y.Z. et al. (2022), 'Understanding associations between rumination and inflammation: a scoping review', *Neuroscience & Behavioral Reviews*, 135, p. 104523. doi: 10.1016/j.neubiorev.2022.104523 **and** Brueckmann, M. et al. (2025), 'Repetitive negative thinking mediates the relationship between self-esteem and burnout in an ecological momentary assessment study', *Communications Psychology*, 3, p.134. doi: 10.1038/s44271-025-00318-2

196 affirming words can potentially enhance inner steadiness, joy and neuroplasticity: Cascio, C.N., O'Donnell, M.B., Tinney, F.J., et al. (2016), 'Self-affirmation activates brain systems associated with self-related processing and reward and is reinforced by future orientation', *Social Cognitive and Affective Neuroscience*, 11(4), pp. 621–629. doi: 10.1093/scan/nsv136

197 positively influence brainwave activity: Bayan, T. and Deb, N., 'Effect of Mantra Chanting on Power Spectral Density', *Indian Journal of Science and Technology*, 2025. **and** Bongarge, K.S. et al., 'A Review of the Effect of Omkar Mantra Chanting on the Nervous System and Its Benefits', *International Journal of Research in Ayurveda and Pharmacy*, 13(3), 2022. **and** Sreenivasan, S., 'The Impact of Vedic Chanting Intervention on Sustained Attention and Working Memory', *International Journal of Indian Psychology*, 12(1), 2024, 269–282.

200 all help build this reserve: Meng, X. and D'Arcy, C., 'Education and Dementia in the Context of the Cognitive Reserve Hypothesis: A Systematic Review with Meta-Analyses and Qualitative Analyses', *PLoS One*, 7(6), 2012, e38268. **and** Asthana, S. et al., 'Occupational Complexity and Cognitive Reserve in a Middle-Aged Cohort at Risk for Alzheimer's Disease', *Archives of Clinical Neuropsychology*, 30(7), November 2015, 634–642. **and** Cheng, S.T., 'Cognitive Reserve and the Prevention of Dementia: The Role of Physical and Cognitive Activities', *Current Psychiatry Reports*, 18(9), September 2016, 85.

201 support more positive perceptions of one's creative abilities: Kaimal, G. et al., 'Functional Near-Infrared Spectroscopy Assessment of Reward Perception Based on Visual Self-Expression: Coloring, Doodling, and Free Drawing', *The Arts in Psychotherapy*, 55, 2017, 85.

201 cognitive decline and dementia: Wu, Z. et al., 'Lifestyle Enrichment in Later Life and Its Association With Dementia Risk', *JAMA Network Open*, 6(7), 2023, e2323690.

201 your brain lighting up, adapting and growing: Lorents, A., Ruitenberg, M.F.L. and Schomaker, J., 'Novelty-Induced Memory Boosts in Humans: The When and How', *Heliyon*, 9(3), 8 March 2023, e14410.

202 purpose, play and lifelong curiosity: Kreouzi, M., Theodorakis, N. and Constantinou, C., 'Lessons Learned From Blue Zones, Lifestyle Medicine Pillars and Beyond: An Update on the Contributions of Behavior and Genetics to Well-Being and Longevity', *American Journal of Lifestyle Medicine*, 18(6), 20 August 2022, 750–765.

202 staying mentally flexible helps protect against cognitive decline: Fastame, M.C., Brandas, B. and Pau, M., 'Is Cognitive Reserve a Determinant of Functional and Mental Health in Older People of the Sardinian Blue Zone? A Mediational Approach', *Psychiatric Quarterly*, 94(4), December 2023, 617–632.

202 linked with higher life expectancy: Bavishi, A., Slade, M.D. and Levy, B.R., 'A Chapter a Day: Association of Book Reading With Longevity', *Social Science & Medicine*, 164, September 2016, 44–48.

203 *svādhyāya* may engage brain networks: Northoff, G., Heinzel, A., de Greck, M., Bermpohl, F., Dobrowolny, H. and Panksepp, J. (2011), 'Self-processing and the default mode network', *Personality and Social Psychology Review*, 15(2), pp. 151–167. https://doi.org/10.1177/1088868310382258 **and** Moore, A. and Malinowski, P. (2009), 'Meditation, mindfulness and cognitive flexibility', *Consciousness and Cognition*, 18(1), pp. 176–186. https://doi.org/10.1016/j.concog.2008.12.008

203 ease the effects of stress on the mind and body: Taren, A.A. et al., 'Mindfulness Meditation Training and Executive Control Network Resting State Functional Connectivity: A Randomized Controlled Trial', *Psychosomatic Medicine*, 79(6), July–August 2017, 674–683. **and** Calderone, A. et al., 'Neurobiological Changes Induced by Mindfulness and Meditation: A Systematic Review', *Biomedicines*, 12(11), 15 November 2024, 2613.

205 mental clarity and emotional balance: Radun, J. et al., 'Speech Is Special: The Stress Effects of Speech, Noise, and Silence During Tasks Requiring Concentration', *Indoor Air*, 31(1), 2021, 264–274.

205 improvements in anxiety, depression and pain: Goyal, M. et al., 'Meditation Programs for Psychological Stress and Well-Being: A Systematic Review and Meta-Analysis', *JAMA Internal Medicine*, 174(3), 2014, 357–368.

205 improving immune function and reducing inflammation: Jamil, A. et al. 'Meditation and Its Mental and Physical Health Benefits in 2023', *Cureus*, 15(6), 19 June 2023, e40650.

205 older adults with moderate sleep disturbances: Tran, E. et al., 'Benefits of Meditation and Breathing Exercises in Vision Loss Patients', *British Journal of Visual Impairment*, 42, 2023, 210–224.

205 increased frontal theta activity (4–8Hz): Tang, Y.Y., Tang, R., Rothbart, M.K. and Posner, M.I. (2019), 'Frontal theta activity and white matter plasticity following mindfulness meditation', *Current Opinion in Psychology*, 28, 294–297. DOI: https://doi.org/10.1016/j.copsyc.2019.04.004

208 walking in natural environments may help reduce inflammation in the body: Kendra, R. and Baldwin, D.R., 'The Effects of Nature Experiences on Inflammation', *Brain, Behavior, and Immunity*, 121, 2024, 176–177.

208 risks of both physical and mental health conditions: Cox, D.T.C. et al., 'Residing in Urban Areas With Higher Green Space Is Associated With Lower Mortality Risk: A Census-Based Cohort Study With Ten Years of Follow-Up', *Environmental Research*, 192, 2021, 110293.

209 You are as young as you feel: Aftab, A. et al., 'Subjective Age and Its Relationships With Physical, Mental, and Cognitive Functioning: A Cross-Sectional Study of 1,004 Community-Dwelling Adults Across the Lifespan', *Journal of Psychiatric Research*, 152, August 2022, 160–166.

210 regularly practise gratitude tend to sleep better: Wood, A.M. et al., 'Gratitude Influences Sleep Through the Mechanism of Pre-Sleep Cognitions', *Journal of Psychosomatic Research*, 66(1), January 2009, 43–48.

Pillar 6

221 Grief, for example, has been shown to depress immune function: Irwin, M. et al., 'Impaired Natural Killer Cell Activity During Bereavement', *Brain, Behavior, and Immunity*, 1(1), 1987, 98–104. **and** O'Connor, M.-F. et al., 'Diurnal Cortisol in Complicated and Non-Complicated Grief: Slope Differences Across the Day', *Psychoneuroendocrinology*, 37(5), 2012, 725–728.

222 boost immunity and even relieve pain: Akimbekov, N.S. and Razzaque, M.S., 'Laughter Therapy: A Humor-Induced Hormonal Intervention to Reduce Stress and Anxiety', *Current Research in Physiology*, 4, 2021, 135–138. **and** Berk, L.S. et al., 'Neuroendocrine and Stress Hormone Changes During Mirthful Laughter', *American Journal of the Medical Sciences*, 298(6), December 1989, 390–396.

222 Research shows clear links to digestive issues (IBS) and headaches: Irwin, M., Daniels, M., Smith, T. L., Bloom, E. and Weiner, H. (1987), 'Impaired natural killer cell activity during bereavement', *Brain, Behavior, and Immunity*, 1(1), 98–104. **and** O'Connor, M.-F., Wellisch, D.K., Stanton, A.L., Eisenberger, N.I., Irwin, M.R. and Lieberman, M.D. (2012), 'Diurnal cortisol in Complicated and Non-Complicated Grief: Slope Differences Across the Day', *Psychoneuroendocrinology*, 37(5), 725–728.

222 Smiling more often can reduce stress: Kraft, T.L. and Pressman, S.D., 'Grin and Bear It: The Influence of Manipulated Facial Expression on the Stress Response', *Psychological Science*, 23(11), 2012, 1372–1378.

222 and lift your spirits: Strack, F., Martin, L.L. and Stepper, S., 'Inhibiting and Facilitating Conditions of the Human Smile: A Nonobtrusive Test of the Facial Feedback Hypothesis', *Journal of Personality and Social Psychology*, 54(5), 1988, 768–777.

227–8 people aged 65-plus lived in care homes in England and Wales: Office for National Statistics, 'Older People Living in Care Homes and Changes Since 2011', 2023.

228 over 350,000 residents in care homes across England: Department of Health & Social Care, 'Adult Social Care in England: Monthly Statistics, August 2025', 2025.

Pillar 7

233 **Data from the Wisconsin Longitudinal Study:** Konrath, S.H., Frazier, S.L., Brown, S.L., Sheridan, J.F. and Kuhlman, D.M. (2012), 'Motives for volunteering are associated with mortality risk in older adults', *Health Psychology*, 31(1), 87–96. DOI: https://doi.org/10.1037/a0025989

233 **protecting us against chronic diseases:** SSM Health, '2022–2024 Community Health Needs Implementation Strategy', *SSM Health*, 2022. Available at: www.ssmhealth.com/SSMHealth/media/Documents/about/chna/illinois/ssm-health-southern-illinois-chip-2022-2024.pdf

239 **opens the door to mental clarity:** Calderone, A., Camacho-Freire, C. and Fraguas, D. (2024), 'Neurobiological changes induced by mindfulness and meditation practices: A systematic review', *Frontiers in Psychiatry*, 15, 1427694.DOI: https://doi.org/10.3389/fpsyt.2024.1427694

239 **reflected in stronger immunity, reduced inflammation:** Katrinli, S., Perlis, R.H. and Binder, E.B. (2022), 'The role of the immune system in posttraumatic stress disorder', *Nature Mental Health*, 1, 588–602. DOI: https://doi.org/10.1038/s41398-022-02094-7

243 **As Anita Moorjani articulates in her book:** Moorjani, A., *Dying to be me: My journey from cancer, to near death, to true healing* (10th anniversary ed.) (Hay House UK Ltd., 2022).

Resources

Global Ayurvedic Practitioner Directories

USA: National Ayurvedic Medical Association (NAMA): www.ayurvedanama.org/
UK: Ayurvedic Practitioners Association UK (APA): apa.uk.com/
UK: British Ayurvedic Medical Council: www.britishayurvedicmedcouncil.com/
EU: European Institute of Vedic Studies: www.eivs.org/
Australia: Australian Ayurveda Association: www.ayurved.org.au/
Canada: Canadian Association of Ayurveda: capassociation.ca/
Portugal: Portuguese Association for Ayurvedic Medicine (AMAYUR) amayur.pt/
Source your own natural spring water: findaspring.org/
Kansa Comb, Kansa Wand, Tongue Scraper: www.geetavara.co.uk/shop

For an extensive live and updated list of *rasāyana* resources go to:
www.geetavara.co.uk/rasayana-resources
or scan the QR code here:

You will find useful websites, product suppliers, recommended further reading and podcasts, retreats and centres, global practitioner directories, further learning and more.

Connect with Geeta

Head to **geetavara.co.uk** for Āyurvedic consultations, coaching, workshops, retreats, courses and workplace wellness
Instagram, YouTube, Threads, LinkedIn: @geetavara

Classical Ayurvedic Scriptures

Bhāvamiśra (1998), *Bhāvaprakāsha of Bhāvamishra: Text, English translation, notes and appendices*. Translated by K.R. Srikantha Murthy. Two vols. Varanasi: Chaukhambha Krishnadas Academy

Charaka (1976–2002), *Charaka Samhitā*. Translated by R.K. Sharma and B. Dash. Seven vols. New Delhi: Chowkhamba Sanskrit Series

Patañjali (1989), *The Yoga Sūtras of Patañjali: A New Edition, Translation, and Commentary*. Translated by Edwin F. Bryant. New York: North Point Press.

Sushruta (1907–1916), *Sushruta Samhitā*. Translated by K.K. Bhishagratna. Three vols. Calcutta. Reprint: Varanasi: Chowkhamba Sanskrit Series

Svātmārāma (2002), *Haṭha Yoga Pradīpikā of Svātmārāma*. Translated by Pancham Sinh. Varanasi: Chaukhambha Sanskrit Series

Tewari, P.V. (2018), *Kāśyapa Saṃhitā, or Vṛddhajīvakiya Tantra*. Edited and translated by P.V. Tewari. Varanasi: Chaukhambha Viśvabharati.

Vāgbhaṭa (1991–1995), *Ashtāṅga Hṛdaya: Text, English translation, notes, appendices and index*. Translated by K.R. Srikantha Murthy. Three vols. Varanasi: Chaukhambha Orientalia

Warrier, A.G. Krishna (trans.) (1981), *The Bhagavad Gītā: With the Commentary of Shrī Shankarācārya*. Madras: Samata Books

Acknowledgements

This book began with a simple promise I made to myself over 20 years ago – to follow what felt true. To walk a path rooted in purpose, however uncertain or unconventional. When I found *Āyurveda* (or rather when it found me), it offered me not just profound wisdom, but a conscious way of life. *Āyurveda* became my compass, my devotion, and the language through which I could finally understand myself and the world.

Writing this book has been both a joy and a challenge. It has been a deeply personal and often solitary process that called for discipline, reflection, passion and deep trust. The knockbacks in 2020, and the growth that followed, could easily have derailed this offering. But in hindsight, perhaps it was simply ahead of its time. So I waited patiently, trusting in divine timing. This book is shaped by persistence, clarity and faith in a natural unfurling.

My heartfelt thanks to my agent, Laetitia Rutherford, for her gentle persistence and unwavering belief. To my wonderful team at Bloomsbury, especially Holly Jarrald, for receiving *Rasayāna* with such warmth and enthusiasm – thank you for holding the vision so delicately from the outset; and my sincere appreciation to Megan Jones for her unwavering patience and invaluable editorial expertise. Much gratitude to the wonderful insights from the survey participants.

To my ancestors, thank you for walking beside me in spirit, for your blessings and for entrusting me to carry this wisdom forward. To the teachers, friends and readers who truly see me – your support is what brings light to this work. To my family, for reminding me what it means to grow, love and become. And to the sanctity of life itself, in all its beauty, mess and mystery, I am humbled and I thank you.

ॐ तत् सत्
Oṃ Tat Sat